Cancer
What it is and how it's treated

GW00802037

Cancer
What it is and how it's treated

Howard Smedley, Karol Sikora
and Rob Stepney

Basil Blackwell

© Howard Smedley, Karol Sikora and Rob Stepney, 1985

First published 1985

Basil Blackwell Ltd
108 Cowley Road, Oxford Ox4 1JF, UK

Basil Blackwell Inc.
432 Park Avenue South, Suite 1505,
New York, NY 10016, USA

British Library in Cataloguing in Publication Data
Smedley, Howard M.
   Cancer: what it is and how it's treated.
   1. Cancer
   I. Title   II. Sikora, Karol   III. Stepney, Rob   616.99′4   RC261

ISBN 0-631-14039-5
ISBN 0-631-14041-7 Pbk

Library of Congress Cataloging in Publication Data
Smedley, Howard M.
   Cancer, what it is and how it's treated.

   Includes index.
   1. Cancer.   I. Sikora, Karol.   II. Stepney, Rob.
III. Title.   [DNLM: 1. Neoplasms—popular works.
QZ 201 S637c]
RC263.S56   1985   616.99′4   85-3937
ISBN 0-631-14039-5
ISBN 0-631-14041-7 (pbk.)

Typeset by Katerprint Co. Ltd, Oxford
Printed in Great Britain by Whitstable Litho, Whitstable, Kent

Contents

About the Authors

Dr Howard Smedley is a Consultant Radiotherapist and Oncologist at the Kent and Canterbury Hospital, Kent. He qualified in medicine at University College Hospital and trained in radiotherapy at Cambridge. He was clinical fellow at the Ludwig Institute for Cancer Research in Cambridge before his present position. His research interests include the clinical application of monoclonal antibodies in oncology and trials of new anti-cancer agents.

Dr Karol Sikora is Director of the Ludwig Institute for Cancer Research, Cambridge and Consultant in Radiotherapy and Oncology at Addenbrooke's and Hinchingbrooke Hospitals. He qualified at Cambridge and the Middlesex Hospital and after various clinical posts in London returned to Cambridge to work in the MRC Laboratory of Molecular Biology. This was followed by senior registrar posts in Cambridge and Stanford, California prior to taking up his present position. His research involves applying recent advances in molecular biology to the diagnosis and treatment of cancer.

Rob Stepney is a freelance medical writer and journalist, with an MA degree in psychology and philosophy from Oxford, an MSc in pharmacology from Newcastle, and a PhD in medicine from Cambridge. He edits a cardiology magazine and was special correspondent for *World Medicine*. He has also contributed material on medicine, science and travel to *The Observer*, *Guardian*,

Sunday Times, *New Scientist*, *New Society* and the BBC. With Heather Ashton, he wrote *Smoking: Psychology and Pharmacology* published last year in paperback by Tavistock/Methuen.

Acknowledgements

The authors thank Susan Hamilton, Mary Smedley, Alison Sikora and Christina Surawy for their help with this book.

Landmarks in our Understanding and Treatment of Cancer

- Ancient Descriptions of tumours   500BC

- First cancer ward (established at the   1792
  Middlesex Hospital London)

- Radical mastectomy for breast cancer   1898

- Viruses shown to cause cancer in animals   1910

- First use of chemotherapy   1945

- Development of high energy radiotherapy   1955
  machines

- First effective combination chemotherapy   1965
  for Hodgkin's disease

- Development of CT scanning   1976

Introduction

From harmless skin warts, to the commonest cause of death in the developed world – cancer has many faces, varying greatly in their features and fatality. One in four of us will at some time have a serious form of the disease. That does not show cancer is getting out of control, or that it is certain death. The simple fact is that as we find cures to other illnesses, the impact made by cancer increases. And that happens even though several forms of the disease can already be very successfully treated.

But the one in four chance means that cancer has become almost everybody's business. Sooner or later, all of us will meet the disease, in ourselves or in our dearest relatives and friends. What should we know about it, and how should we react?

Recently there have been great advances in our knowledge of what causes cancer, and encouraging progress in its cure. There are computerised scanners to take X-ray sections of the body, and techniques using radioactivity to find hidden cancers. Complicated combinations of drugs kill tumour cells, often with great success, whilst radiotherapy is increasingly sophisticated in its ability to hit cancers without harming the healthy tissue that surrounds them. Surgery no longer means inevitably disfiguring operations. And we are on the threshold of being able to strengthen parts of the body's own defence system, and harness them as powerful new tools for diagnosing and treating the disease. It is a revolution which will do for medicine what the silicon chip has done for electronics.

There is still unnecessary fear and misunderstanding about cancer, though much progress has been made and the subject is no longer taboo. In this book, two doctors experienced in treating cancer patients and in cancer research present a scientific and humane approach.

The growth in popularity of alternative 'treatments' shows that many people have been dissatisfied with what doctors offer. Part of the problem is that patients do not always have the information needed to participate in the decisions that are made. An increasingly aware public rightly demands to understand the disease more fully and to have the complicated costs and benefits of different courses of treatment clearly presented.

Cancer is the biggest challenge faced by the medical scientist. That the disease has not yet been overcome does not show the medical approach is wrong. We now advance from a sure basis of knowledge, and have treatments of proven worth. If we are to find a way of finally overcoming cancer it must be to the laboratory that we look for a more complete understanding of the disease.

But this is not a specialist text. It explains the cancer problem in non-technical language. The first two chapters present our scientific understanding of the basis of cancer, its causes, and effects on the patient. Then diagnostic techniques are described, together with the way the information they provide is used in deciding the best form of treatment. Several common cancers are discussed in depth, and conventional methods of treatment – surgery, radiotherapy and the use of drugs – assessed. The impact of widely- publicised alternative approaches to cancer is covered, and the book ends with a glimpse of the cancer medicine we are likely to see by the end of the century.

1 What is Cancer?

The cell is the basic building block of our bodies. All our tissues and organs are made up of them. In an average sized person there are around one thousand billion; and cancer can start in any one. The disease is not easy to treat: it is not even easy to describe. But in simplest terms it is the continual, uncontrolled production of cells that are of no benefit to the body. In most cases, as the cells proliferate, they form a swelling. 'Tumour' is originally just another word for this.

Such swellings or 'growths' have been recognised since the time of the ancient Greeks. It was discovered very early in medical history that if one of the swellings was removed and cut open, it had a very typical appearance: a central area and then channels of spread, like arms, as the rapidly dividing cells which are already squashed closely together start to invade healthy tissue. This was thought to look something like a crab – hence use of the word 'cancer', Latin for crab, to describe the growth. Cancer is also referred to as 'neoplasm', from the Greek 'new growth'.

The word 'cancer' can also be used in cases where there is abnormal proliferation of cells, but no swelling. This happens when the blood-forming cells are affected, producing diseases known as the leukaemias and lymphomas.

Why should the simple fact that there are too many cells cause such harm? The problem lies not just in their number, but in the fact that cancer cells also change their nature. For individual species, evolution is a process of more and more precise adaptation to a particular environment; for the cell it is one of increasing specialisation. Normally cells perform a specific function; the particular job they do depending on the organ they belong to. Liver cells, for example, purify the blood by removing toxic chemicals; muscle cells provide mechanical power. But once cells start to grow wildly, this specialism is lost. Instead of doing a job useful to the organism as a whole, they become independent entities, seeking nutrition and support wherever they can, often at the expense of normal healthy tissue.

Even with this feature, the problem of cancer would still be manageable, but for the fact that cancer often spreads to parts of the body far removed from the original tumour. Cells break off the parent growth and are carried away in the stream of blood or tissue fluid to set up new tumours wherever they happen to settle. Such dispersion of cancer is termed secondary, or metastatic, growth.

Cancers which spread in this way are called 'malignant', and the terms 'malignancy' and 'cancer' are often used interchangeably. But it should be remembered that not all cancers are malignant. Some cells, though they start to divide unnecessarily quickly, still reproduce at a relatively slow rate and tend to stay in one place in the body. Such localised tumours are called benign. Despite this, they can have serious consequences. If the swelling produced is in a confined space, such as within the skull, the tumour can block blood vessels and compress nerves. But such comparatively innocent growths can usually be removed completely, in which case they do not recur. The most important differences between benign and malignant growths are shown in figure 1.1.

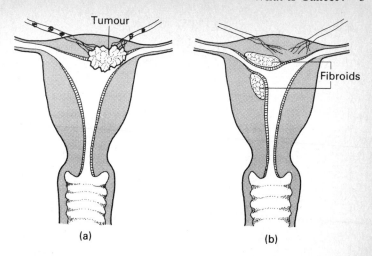

Figure 1.1 (a) A malignant tumour of the body of the uterus. The cancer has an irregular, ulcerated surface. There is no capsule enclosing it, and the tumour is invading the normal tissue that surrounds it. Some of the malignant cells break off and are carried away in the bloodstream. In this way, the cancer can spread to other parts of the body. (b) Benign tumours of the uterus, such as fibroids, are smooth in appearance and contained in a capsule. The tumour grows slowly and does not invade surrounding tissue. There can be symptoms (heavy periods, for example, and pain) but there is no danger that the disease will spread to other organs.

Cells growing out of control

So small that they can only be seen under a microscope, each cell is a complex biological factory. At its heart, lies the nucleus – its control centre. If the nucleus of one cell is taken out and the nucleus of a different cell returned in its place, the recipient cell will change its structure and function to behave as the new nucleus directs. Rather as in a computer, the nucleus contains all the information needed for the cell's proper functioning. This information is in the form of the molecule DNA, the famous double-

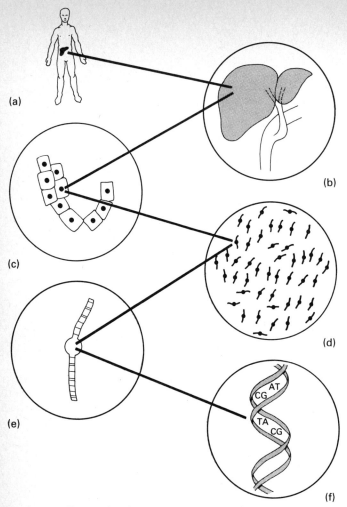

Figure 1.2 *The Scale of Things*. The body (a) showing the size and position of the liver – one of our many organs. The liver itself (b) is composed of millions of cells (c), each with a central nucleus (d) containing 46 chromosomes (e) and hundreds of thousands of genes (which can be made to appear as bands) containing DNA – the blueprint of life. DNA (f) is made up of infinitely variable sequences of the four chemical building blocks called A, C, T and G. Certain rearrangements of these building blocks can lead to cancer.

helix discovered thirty years ago in Cambridge by Watson and Crick. (See figure 1.2.)

Fundamental to our understanding of cancer is the fact that each cell in the body contains the same inherited, genetic information as every other cell. When it is remembered that they all come ultimately from one fertilised egg – which is itself a single cell – this is not so difficult to understand. But the fact that cells perform such different functions makes it seem surprising. They do different jobs only because in any one cell at any time the great bulk of the genetic information is firmly switched off.

In normal healthy tissue, each cell has a limited life-span. Cells constantly die, or are lost, and so must be replaced. New cells are also needed to accommodate growth. In a developing child, for example, they have to be laid down in the bone and skin. To produce them, existing cells divide into two. This also happens after injury, when cells next to the wound reproduce more quickly to repair the damage. But this process is normally tightly controlled so that it operates only when the body needs new tissue. Once growth is complete, the rate of cell division is reduced. And when an injury is repaired it is somehow recognised that healing has occurred and the extra division of cells stops.

Cancerous change produces a cell that continues to divide; one that is unable to recognise when such division is no longer necessary.

Mapping cancer spread

As the initial cancer grows, it interferes with the working of healthy tissue that surrounds it. In spreading to other parts of the body it repeats the process wherever migrating tumour cells take root. These secondary cancers are just as dangerous as the parent tumour. A secondary tumour growing in bone weakens its mechanical strength so that even a normal amount of physical pressure can cause the bone to break. This is how the existence of some

cancers is first recognised. In colonising the brain, lungs
or liver – which are all likely to pick up wandering cancer
cells because of the large volume of blood that passes
through – secondary growths interfere with the normal
function of these organs and can themselves cause
symptoms.

In treating cancer, the essence of the problem is to
determine first of all the exact extent of disease, and this
means looking for evidence of the tumour far beyond the
site where the primary cancer was found. Treatment of a
small tumour confined to one organ of the body will be
very different from treatment of a cancer that has already
spread widely. There are also implications for the chances
of cure. In the majority of cases a primary tumour can be
successfully treated using existing methods. But widespread dissemination of disease often causes treatment to
fail. For this reason, the importance of early diagnosis is
stressed. Catch a cancer before it has had time to spread
and the outlook is much brighter. Here, screening clinics,
to detect the earliest stages of cancer in apparently healthy people, may help.

Why this enemy within?

The fact that cells become malignant, putting at risk the
life of the organism of which they are a part, is something
of a biological mystery. When parasites, or micro-
organisms (like bacteria and viruses) cause disease it is
easy enough to see this contest as just another round in an
evolutionary battle in which different forms of life 'prey'
on each other. But in cancer it is the cells of our own
bodies which seem to rebel against us. Why should we
have built into us a process with such potential for going
disastrously wrong?

When an apparent disadvantage occurs, the biologist
looks for a reason why, in the long run, it may benefit the
individual. There is a type of anaemia which provides a
good example. Certain abnormalities of the oxygen-

carrying blood pigment haemoglobin cause severe anaemia, with attendant weakness and debility. But the abnormalities somehow also confer protection against malaria, and are found mostly in parts of the world where malaria is a life-threatening disease.

But a process which threatens so many of us with malignant disease could have no survival advantage. It looks like a fundamental biological error. Why then has the susceptibility to cancer not been weeded out along the evolutionary way? What causes an individual cell to reverse millions of years of evolution and revert to a primitive undifferentiated state? Malignant disease occurs in all orders of animals and plants, suggesting that the process that gives rise to it is very basic to life. This idea is explored in the chapter on the causes of cancer.

Cancer and age

A cell is made cancerous by a particular kind of change occurring in its genetic material. It is likely that one of the times such a change can occur is when the cell divides. So the number of times a cell has reproduced is some indication of the risk of it becoming cancerous. In older people, cells have undergone many more divisions, and the chance that a malignant transformation has taken place somewhere along the line is therefore greater. Apart from a few rare and special kinds of tumour, cancer is increasingly common with age.

It follows that as the number of people surviving to old age increases, the incidence of cancer in the population will also increase. The fact that one person in five in the western world now dies of cancer does not mean that the environmental causes of the disease are more common. Neither does it show our efforts to treat the disease are always ineffectual. It simply means that fewer people are dying of other diseases. And the obvious reasons for that are the changes in hygiene and nutrition, plus the development of antibiotics, which have eliminated much infectious illness. The decline in tuberculosis as a cause of death, particularly in young people, is a prime example.

Different kinds of cancer

Tumours can occur in any organ of the body. Many of the features which set their parent cell apart as coming from a particular organ are lost in the development of the disease; and of course cancers have often spread far from their original site. But it is still usual for tumours to be classified by the place they originated, and this can be established by examining a specimen of the cancerous tissue under the microscope. A tumour which starts in the breast, for example, continues to be called breast cancer, even though the tumour cells may be found in the brain or bone. The original site is known as the primary, and the far-flung colonies metastatic breast cancer.

This classification is useful because careful study of large numbers of cases shows that cancers originating in a certain tissue often behave in particular and predictable ways. Malignant tumours that start in the salivary glands, for example, are very slow to grow, even if they have spread in other organs. It is also known that in three-quarters of patients with primary lung cancer, the disease has spread beyond the volume of lung that can safely be removed by surgery before the disease is advanced enough to cause symptoms. This usual course of development of a cancer is termed its natural history. Such knowledge is a useful guide. It suggests which parts of the body should be investigated to see if secondary spread has occurred, and allows the chances of cure to be estimated.

The natural history of a disease is also vital to the planning of treatment. Leukaemia, a cancer of the blood affecting both children and adults, is a good example. When anti-cancer drugs became available, it was possible to clear the patients' blood of malignant cells. But many patients went on to develop disease within the brain and the fluid that surrounds it and the spinal cord (cerebro-spinal fluid). Because of this observation, many people with leukaemia now have drugs injected into the cere-brospinal fluid even if they show no signs of disease there at the time. This treatment of what are termed 'sanctuary' sites has led to a great improvement in the rate of cure.

Tumours arising from similar tissues within the body tend to have a particular name, as is shown in table 1.1. Probably the largest group of malignancies, including those of the skin, stomach, bowel and breast, is termed 'carcinomas'. These cancers have in common the fact that they start in cells which form the linings of body surfaces, internal and external. (Such cells are called epithelial.) Tumours arising from the body's structural tissues, such as muscle, bone and tendons, are known as 'sarcomas'.

Connective tissues

Table 1.1 Cancers are described not only by the organ where they start (the stomach or lung, for example) but also by the type of tissue from which they originate.

Type of tissue where tumour originates	General name of tumour
Epithelial tissue e.g.: colon, skin or lung	Carcinoma
Connective tissue e.g.: muscle, fat, bone	Sarcoma
Blood cells	Leukaemia
Lymphatic system	Lymphoma

How cancer damages the body

Cancers can cause local problems in the part of the body where they form, *and* have more widespread effects. In both cases the severity of the symptoms which result depends on the kind of tumour and the particular organ involved.

In the case of both benign and malignant growths, the size of the tumour itself is the most obvious source of difficulties. Normal tissue, under increasing pressure from the tumour, may become damaged and die. The expansion of a tumour is particularly dangerous if a large artery is compressed, since interrupting the flow of oxygenated blood can cause the death of wide areas of the body which the artery serves. The growth of a mass within the brain is especially serious, since the skull is rigid and prevents expansion. Increase in size of the tumour can therefore only be at the expense of normal tissue.

Invasion and erosion

With malignant tumours, the problem is not just one of a mass of cancer cells occupying space and pressing on normal tissue. The cells' prodigious capacity for growth means that they actually invade and erode local tissue, disrupting its organisation and function. Certain types of lung tumour, for example, may grow directly into the chest wall surrounding the lung and cause pain as nerves are affected. In a similar way, breast tumours left untreated can break through the skin, causing an ulcer.

A particular feature of malignant tumours is their ability to erode even bone, the hardest of body tissues. Cancer cells do this by secreting substances that dissolve the calcium of which bone is made, and by obstructing arteries that supply the bone with nutrients.

Secretion also holds the key to understanding how cancer has such widespread effects, since, as well as disrupting the body by direct contact with healthy tissue, malignant tumours also act at a distance.

Abnormal hormone production

Many of the body's processes are controlled by substances secreted into the bloodstream by particular organs. Prime examples of these chemical messengers are the hormones, produced by specialised cells in the endocrine glands, such as the thyroid. As we have seen, tumours are formed of primitive cells in which the mechanisms that control the production of certain chemicals no longer function. This means that a tumour cell can manufacture many substances which its parent cell would not normally produce. Among them are hormones which are chemically identical to those manufactured by the specialist endocrine glands. These tumour products are not in themselves toxic. But symptoms occur because the amounts produced exceed the body's requirements.

Although at some time or other most hormones have been found to be produced by most tumours, certain common associations are known. These include the ability of certain types of lung cancer to produce hormones normally manufactured in the pituitary gland which increase blood pressure and cause kidney disorders and weakness of the muscles. Other tumours secrete a hormone which in excess leads to abnormally high calcium levels in the body, and symptoms of nausea, thirst and constipation. Cancers can also produce hormones that make the body retain water but excrete salt, and this imbalance causes psychiatric symptoms.

There are other rarer, but striking examples. Tumours of the testis have been known to produce enough female hormones to stimulate breast development and for a pregnancy test to prove positive. There are also tumours of the ovaries which secrete sufficient testosterone, the male hormone, to lead to growth of facial hair.

Loss of energy and weight
The widespread systemic effects of cancer can cause anything from skin rashes to hallucinations. But there are two very common features of advanced disease: a general feeling and appearance of being unwell, and weight loss.

In sustaining themselves, tumour cells may cause the body to become deficient in vital elements such as iron. This in turn leads to anaemia, characterised by tiredness and lack of energy. Anaemia is also produced by under-activity of the patient's marrow, a substance which lies at the centre of most bones and which is responsible for the production of blood. Bone marrow is very sensitive to general well-being, and so – among other things – to the presence of cancer. Its suppression also leads to an increased likelihood of infection, and so to further debilitating effects.

These are certain of the reasons cancer patients feel unwell, and they can be understood and treated. But it seems the presence of cancer itself may cause people to feel profoundly ill. We still do not know why. It is possible to correct anaemia and vitamin deficiency, and protect patients from infection, and still have them feel terribly unwell.

Weight loss is also difficult to explain fully. But again it is a very sensitive indicator of the presence of cancer. A patient who has recently and unintentionally lost weight may have no specific symptoms of a recurrence of the tumour, yet the mere fact of weight loss is sufficient to alert the physician. Even if calorie intake is maintained, a patient with an active tumour is still likely to lose weight. This observation has led to the search for substances secreted by tumours which may be the cause. Over the past 20 years, several laboratories have claimed they have identified specific weight-losing factors in the blood serum of cancer patients, but nothing has been satisfactorily proved.

It is particularly hard to account for the fact that weight loss selectively affects healthy tissue. The tumours themselves continue to grow even as patients weaken, so it would appear that they have a preferential hold over the body's reserves of energy. However primitive the biochemical processes going on in cancer cells, they are clearly very successful.

2   The Causes of Cancer

Much is made of factors in the environment that may be responsible for cancer. The most recent authoritative estimates suggest that up to 80 per cent of cases are due to causes that are environmental in the broad sense of the term – that is, including diet, lifestyle, specific habits such as smoking, as well as exposure in the workplace. This implies that a great many cancers could be prevented. But there is no single change in our environment or lifestyle which would reduce the incidence of all forms of cancer.

Just as there are many types of cancer, so there are many causes. The range of factors involved includes physical agents such as heat, continual irritation, and radiation (which encompasses ultraviolet light from the sun); chemical agents like those found in cigarette smoke and in certain of the foods we eat; and viruses.

If a cell is damaged in such a way that it dies, no cancer can result. That cell is deleted from the population, and cannot reproduce. The problem arises with cells that have been damaged to the extent that the mechanism controlling their growth is no longer effective. This switch from restrained growth to cancerous proliferation may be sudden. But it is more likely that there is an accumulation of damage, caused by chance events, over a lifetime. At some unpredictable point, the balance tips in favour of malignant growth.

Work using cells grown in the laboratory, and experiments involving animals, suggest that causing a cancer may be a two-stage process, with some factors initiating a cancerous alteration in the genetic material inside a cell nucleus, and others later promoting cell growth. The two crucial events, initiation and promotion, could in theory be years apart. This idea may help explain why some cancers develop only ten or 20 years after exposure to a cause such as uncontrolled radiation. But no-one has ever observed these crucial events taking place. The distinction between initiating and promoting agents is far from clear cut, and there seem to be many other factors involved. So, in accounting for the development of cancer in man, it is probably easier to think simply in terms of the random accumulation of damage over a long period.

This damage consists of alterations in small segments of the DNA genetic code that controls all aspects of cell function. Many sections of DNA can be tampered with without producing malignant change. But there are obviously certain sites that are critical. We are now beginning to find out where these sites are, and how damage to them leads to cancer. But that is the most recent aspect of our understanding, deriving from the sophisticated science of molecular biology. Our first clues about the causes of cancer came from studying the rates of disease in different groups of people: the science of epidemiology.

Clues from patterns of disease

Think for a moment about the people you know who have had a heart attack. Are they similar in any respect? Do they differ as a group from people of the same age who do not have heart disease? It is probably difficult to find anything about the jobs they do, or the way they live, or the kind of personality they have that gives any clues about the origin of the disease. This is because there are many contributory causes, and the pattern is hard to discern. It is only by collecting large amounts of information about hundreds of people that we can begin to see there are certain characteristics – such as obesity, a family history of heart disease, lack of exercise and smoking – that increase the likelihood an individual will suffer from heart disease.

With cancer, there are certain causes which we now take for granted. Smoking and lung cancer is the most obvious example. But even that association was not clear at first. It was only by systematically collecting information on rates of the disease and carefully relating them to differences in smoking habits that the link was established. For the majority of cancers, we still have no clearly identified causes. To help find them, many countries now have a cancer registry. The aim is that records are kept of everyone who develops the disease. Any pattern should then be easier to see. The register is likely to be more reliable than using death certificates, since there are now many cancers that are curable, and the certified cause of death is often open to debate.

The number of people developing cancer in any year is termed the incidence. This is usually expressed as the number of cases that occur for every 100,000 people in the population. Some cancers are relatively common. With breast cancer, the incidence is around 80 per 100,000 women per year. Cancer of the small intestine, on the other hand, at less than one per 100,000 per year, is extremely rare.

It is crucial that accurate information is collected, and expressed in a standard way. Only by doing this can pressing questions be answered. For example, when the alarm was raised about the risk of cancer from nuclear power stations, epidemiologists needed to establish the incidence of cancer among the people who lived near the power stations, and then compare it with the incidence for the population as a whole. The debate over the role of nuclear power stations continues (though the latest evidence suggests there are no real grounds for concern). But picking out regional variations in cancer incidence is a vital help in identifying causes of certain forms of the disease, and has already proved its worth on many occasions.

A notable example is cancer of the oesophagus (the tube connecting the mouth to the stomach), which was reported to be especially common among nomadic tribes living on the high desert plateau near the border between Iran and Afghanistan. In the 1970s, a team of investigators sent by the World Health Organisation established that the disease was indeed the most frequent cause of death among the nomads. The researchers collected samples of urine, faeces and blood from the affected tribes, and also from a comparable population of nomads who lived in the south of Iran and who did not show an elevated incidence of the cancer. Simple laboratory analysis demonstrated that the urine and faeces of the northern nomads contained large quantities of chemicals which damage the DNA of cells. It was soon established that these cancer-causing chemicals (carcinogens) came from a particular process of smoking meat. At least for the Iranian nomads, the cause of oesophageal cancer had been clearly identified.

In Uganda, a very different cause of a very different type of cancer was found by similar epidemiological detective work. In 1960, the missionary surgeon Denis Burkitt began to wonder about the high incidence of a rare type of cancer of the lymphatic system. The pattern of disease was different from that in western countries. First, it occurred mostly in children, often under the age of ten. Secondly, the areas of the body in which the disease made itself apparent – the jaw, kidneys and ovaries – were sites that were not usually involved in patients in the developed world.

It became clear that the geographical distribution of that particular variant of the disease (now known as Burkitt's lymphoma) closely matched that of the Anopheles mosquito, the carrier of malaria. At the same time, laboratory investigation showed that tissues taken from children with the disease contained a micro-organism, the Epstein-Barr virus.

It is now clear that development of the cancer involves several causes acting together. First is the infection of the young child with malaria. The body's immune defences are able to prevent death from the disease, but the persistence of the malarial parasite means that the immune system is in a state of continuous activity. Cells forming part of that system (the lymphocytes) are always dividing, and the spleen, an organ where they are produced, is much enlarged. The second cause is the virus. In normal circumstances, it is unlikely to precipitate cancerous change. But acting against the background of a stimulated immune system, and in the context of general malnutrition, it is sufficient to produce an incidence of Burkitt's lymphoma which is a thousand times greater than that found, for example, in Britain.

In the hope of preventing the disease, African children are now being vaccinated against the Epstein-Barr virus. This is one example of the practical value of epidemiological studies. Unfortunately, most epidemiological insights are not so easily translated into preventive measures. The case of smoking is a prime example. Even when the cause of a cancer can be definitely established, it is not so easy to change deeply ingrained social habits; the same applies in cases where particular diets have been implicated in disease. We also have to face the fact that the origin of many cancers is much more complicated, the factors involved much more general, and at least some of the causes probably beyond our control.

Physical causes

We are surrounded by different forms of energy: movement, heat, light and a range of electromagnetic radiation. Growing cells can be damaged by any of them. But physical agents can also have an important indirect effect simply by increasing the rate at which cells divide. Cancer can probably arise spontaneously, by the occurrence of a random fault during the copying of DNA which precedes cell division. Any factor which leads to faster turnover of cells increases the risk such a fault will occur. One example is continual abrasion: the constant movement of a piece of shrapnel in an old wound, for instance, leads to cell growth as the body attempts to exclude the foreign object. Cancer can occur in the wound site. It also occasionally develops in regenerating tissue at the edge of burns.

In the elderly, it is common for the blood supply to the leg to be impaired. Because of this, any sore that develops heals only slowly, and may produce a shallow ulcer lasting for years – especially if the wound is continually being knocked and reopened. Around the rim of such ulcers, where repair of tissue is being attempted over a long period, there is again a small risk that a cancerous change will take place.

Excessive heat, too, can lead to tumours. People who live in the Tibetan mountains attempt to protect themselves from the bitter cold by placing a small wicker basket, containing embers, next to their skin. This often leads to the formation of cancers on the abdomen, as cells are damaged by a combination of heat and constant rubbing.

It is well known that radiation can cause, as well as cure, cancer. In large enough doses, the DNA double-helix is destroyed, and cells die. But smaller doses simply damage the DNA, including those parts that restrict cell growth. The most horrific example of radiation damage is of course the epidemic of cancer that followed the man-made disasters of Hiroshima and Nagasaki. In the few years immediately following the bombings, there seemed to be no long-term effects. But then acute leukaemias began to appear in excessive numbers among the survivors. Later, the incidence of thyroid cancers rose; and more recently the delayed effects of radiation have been seen in the dramatic increase in breast cancer. The incidence of cancer among survivors is directly related to the distance they were from the centre of the explosion, and so to the amount of radiation they received.

It is not so often realised that there are entirely natural radiation sources that are a significant factor in cancer. Ultraviolet light from the sun's rays is a pervasive form of radiation that can be particularly damaging, as is shown by the fact that agricultural workers in sunny climates often develop skin tumours on exposed parts of the body. We are also bombarded with radiation from space. To some extent, the atmosphere protects us against cosmic radiation. But the dangers it can pose are appreciated by astronauts who experience twice the level of radiation found on earth. When there are solar flares, radiation exposure increases still further, and astronauts carry special drugs to protect them against its effects.

Naturally radioactive minerals deep within the earth also contribute to the background radiation to which we are all exposed. Background levels have increased over the past 30 years, because of the atmospheric testing of nuclear weapons. But with the switch to underground testing these levels are now beginning to fall.

Under normal circumstances, it is unlikely that nuclear power stations will significantly raise our exposure to radiation. But the possibility of accidental release of radioactive materials, with consequent increase in cancer risk, cannot be excluded. Our one safeguard is that the dangers of radiation are now well appreciated. Ranging from the simplest mobile X-ray device to the most complicated defence installation, precautions to prevent unnecessary exposure are stringent.

Chemical causes

Of the millions of chemical compounds that come into contact with our skin, or that are found in the air we breathe and the food we eat, hundreds – perhaps thousands – have the ability to damage DNA in a way that leads to cancer. These chemicals are called carcinogens.

The first suggestion of a link between cancer and occupational exposure to particular substances appeared over two centuries ago. In 1775, Percival Pott, a surgeon at London's St Bartholomew's Hospital, noticed that boys who swept chimneys for a living had a very high incidence of cancer of the scrotum (the sack of skin around the testes). When the chimney sweeps were required by law to wash more regularly, the risk of cancer fell.

Pott made the connection between soot and cancer, but it was not until the early part of this century that we realised the cause lay in chemical carcinogens. Their effects were first demonstrated at the Institute of Cancer Research in London by painting the skin of mice with coal tar obtained from the nearby Fulham Gas Works. The variety of tumours produced set off the search for the specific constituents of coal tar that were responsible.

Individual carcinogenic chemicals were identified, and there was much excitement in the 1920s that the discovery of their structure would lead to a complete understanding of how cancer is caused. But, 60 years on, we still do not understand why certain chemicals produce cancer and others which have a similar structure do not.

The link between specific chemical carcinogens and a naturally occurring form of human cancer was not established until the 1950s, when questionnaires given to patients with lung cancer suggested that risk of developing the disease was greatly increased by cigarette smoking.

The evidence of an association between lung cancer and smoking was not proof that smoking caused the cancer. It remained possible that people at high risk of contracting lung cancer – for reasons entirely unrelated to smoking – just happened to be more likely to smoke. What was needed was a study showing that people who were already smokers, but then gave up, reduced their lung cancer risk.

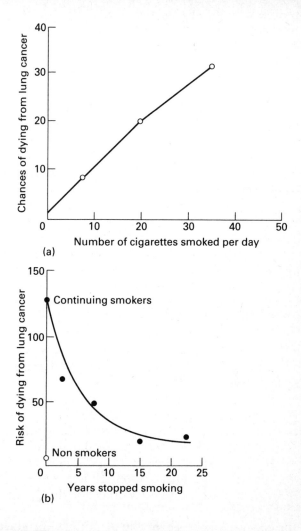

Figure 2.1 The risk of lung cancer increases steadily with the number of cigarettes smoked (a) and starts to decrease as soon as someone stops smoking (b).

The Oxford epidemiologist, Richard Doll, found such a group of people among doctors. Many had been impressed by the early evidence implicating smoking in disease, and so quit the habit. When this group was studied it became clear that there were fewer cases of lung cancer than among those who continued to smoke. In people who gave up, the relative risk of lung cancer started to fall and by 15 years was back at the level of non-smokers. The relationship between smoking and lung cancer, and the beneficial effect of giving up, are shown in figure 2.

Conclusive evidence that smoking caused the disease came also from laboratory work. Tar taken from cigarette smoke was shown to produce cancer when it was painted onto mouse skin. And specific chemicals known to be carcinogenic were identified in cigarette smoke. These chemicals are deposited in the large airways, or bronchi, as they enter the lungs. Over many years, cells lining the airways become damaged, eventually producing cancer in a proportion of smokers. Given the clear evidence that cigarettes cause the disease, it is quite extraordinary that most governments still allow them to be advertised. It is even more scandalous that cigarette promotion linking smoking with healthy activities such as sport is permitted.

Smoking is a clearly preventable cause of disease. But it should be remembered that some of the chemical carcinogens produced by burning tobacco are also found in industrial smoke pollution, and even in the aromatic smoke from garden bonfires. There are also substances such as asbestos that cause particular forms of lung cancer. If no-one smoked cigarettes, the number of cases of lung cancer would fall to about 10 per cent of current levels. However, the disease would not disappear completely.

Lung cancer is a good example of a disease produced by a chemical carcinogen. But there are several other cases where malignant diseases have been linked to chemical exposure. At the turn of the century, a German surgeon who specialised in the treatment of diseases of the urinary system noticed that several patients with bladder cancer came from the same factory. But the great number of processes and substances used at the factory, which made dyes for paints, made it impossible to identify the precise source of the hazard.

It was left to the epidemiologist Robert Case to sort the problem out. From a careful study of factory records throughout Britain between 1920 and 1950, he was able to demonstrate that exposure to aniline dyes was the cause of the increased cancer risk. (Such dyes are widely used in softening rubber for the manufacture of tyres, for example.) Aniline compounds become concentrated in the bladder, where they are changed into a potent carcinogen. The discovery led to the enforced wearing of protective clothing, since when the rate of bladder cancer among rubber workers has returned to that of the general population.

There was a time when the only way of demonstrating that a chemical was carcinogenic was to feed it to animals in large quantities, or inject it under their skin, and see if tumours developed. This caused suffering to animals which can now be avoided. It was also a time-consuming procedure, which meant that few chemicals could be tested. Screening has been greatly helped by the discovery of certain bacteria, related to typhoid, that have a high rate of mutation when exposed to carcinogens. This development, which we owe to the Californian scientist Bruce Ames, means that we can now test large numbers of substances.

From the analysis of urine and faeces it has now become clear that our food contains many chemicals that are themselves possible carcinogens, or that can be changed into carcinogens by digestive enzymes in the stomach and intestines. Some foods contain relatively large quantities. These include barbecued and smoked meats, sausages, and many foods which are preserved.

Work is now in progress to see if slight modifications in the way food is processed, stored and cooked can reduce our exposure to these substances.

There are also studies which hope to relate changes in our diet to decreased risk of disease. Perhaps the chances of developing colon cancer, for example, can be reduced by increasing the amount of fibre that we eat, and decreasing the amount of fat. But it will probably be many years before any firm conclusions can be drawn. The United States National Cancer Institute has committed itself to halving the incidence of cancer by the year 2000. That is going to be an uphill struggle.

Genetic causes

Is cancer inherited? Do the children of parents with cancer have an increased risk of developing the disease? These questions are often asked. In most cases, the answer is No. Cancer is a disease in which accumulated damage to cells eventually triggers a random event leading to the malignant transformation of a cell. It is a kind of shuffling of the genetic cards that eventually produces an unlucky hand. Ultimately, it is a problem in the genes that causes the disease. But it is the genes within a specific cell, rather than within the individual as a whole, that become disordered. However, there are a few exceptions.

In certain relatively rare forms of the disease, the genes inherited by an individual seem to be particularly susceptible to cancerous change: the deck is stacked in favour of a tumour developing. One example is a skin disease called xeroderma pigmentosum. Here, there is an inherited defect in an enzyme that repairs damaged DNA. As children with this condition grow older, damage caused by exposure to the sun's ultraviolet light leads to the development of abnormal patches of skin, some of which eventually become malignant.

There is also what is known as a 'cancer family syndrome', where several members of the family develop cancer, but usually of different types. Presumably there is an inherited defect in some part of a general DNA repair mechanism. This increases the likelihood that any organ may develop cancer when it is exposed to chemical or physical carcinogens. We do not yet know at a molecular level what the repair mechanism is like.

With breast cancer, the relationship to heredity must be slightly different to that found with other common malignant conditions. If several close relatives have had the disease, the chance of other female members of the family developing it is increased three or four-fold. Because of this, the women at risk are given regular clinical examinations and screened with low-power X-rays (a technique called mammography) to detect any disease at an early and more easily curable stage.

Viruses

Viruses can produce cancer in man and animals. Though the number of human cancers they cause may be fairly small, the way they exert their carcinogenic effect has taught us more about the processes that underlie all forms of cancer than study of physical and chemical agents has ever done. Viruses have provided the key to our understanding of the genetic basis of the disease.

Viruses are the simplest form of life. They are basically just a single piece of DNA: a collection of genes, protected by a protein coat. Because the virus does not possess the other structures normally found in cells, it does not have the machinery to build proteins, and so cannot reproduce on its own. To do this it needs to invade a host cell.

The virus attaches itself to the cell membrane and then transfers its genes inside. Once there, the virus starts to act like a cuckoo in the nest. Its genes incorporate themselves into the DNA of the host cell and take it over, so that instead of producing copies of itself, the host cell starts step by step to produce copies of the viral genetic material. The virus genes also instruct the host cell to produce their protective coats so that, after a while, a complete new set of virus particles is formed. These then emerge and move on to infect other cells.

The similarity between the virus genes and those of the host cell makes it possible for the virus to incorporate fragments of the host genes within its own genetic material. These randomly 'snipped out' bits of host gene are then taken to a new cell that the virus infects, where they can combine with that cell's genes. Sometimes this virus-induced exchange of genetic material can be disastrous, damaging a host cell's growth control mechanisms and turning a previously normal cell into one which reproduces wildly to form a tumour. This process is described in greater detail in the section below on cancer genes.

We have known for 70 years that certain viruses cause cancer in animals, including pets such as cats and hamsters; but it is only over the past decade that we have been sure this happens also in man. Though there is little evidence that any of the common human tumours are caused by viruses, they seem to be involved in at least some cancers. We have seen there is evidence linking the Epstein-Barr virus to Burkitt's lymphoma. It is also clear that infection with this same virus causes a tumour of the nasal passages though this effect seems (for reasons unknown) to be confined to people from the Far East.

Cancer of the cervix is also associated with viral infection. It has recently been shown that wart viruses can be isolated from such tumours; and that the number of viral DNA pieces found relates to the likelihood the cancer will invade healthy tissue and spread.

More recently still, a virus has been found to cause a rare form of leukaemia in which a small group of white cells called the T-lymphocytes becomes malignant. The virus is known as the human T-cell leukaemia virus, or HTLV for short. The HTLV virus is also implicated in the development of AIDS (the Acquired Immune Deficiency syndrome), an unusual and often fatal disease in which

the body's defensive immune response becomes ineffective. Though not in itself a malignancy, AIDS often leads
to the development of the otherwise rare skin cancer,
Kaposi's sarcoma. Particularly at risk of contracting the
disease are homosexuals, hard drug addicts, and patients
(such as haemophiliacs) who are frequently transfused
with blood or blood products. It seems that the virus
responsible is transmitted in blood or body secretions.

Cancer genes

There is no doubt that viruses can cause cancer in man
and animals. But since the diseases caused tend to be
uncommon, our discovery of the viral connection is of
only limited practical help. Much more important is the
fact that study of these viruses has given us vital insights
into exactly what goes wrong when a cell becomes cancerous. We are finally beginning to see that the various very
different causes of cancer exert their effects through a
similar mechanism: they have a final common pathway.

At a crucial stage in evolution, probably around a
thousand million years ago, multi-cellular forms of life
developed out of the single-celled organisms that are our
ultimate ancestors. Biologically, this development presented immense problems. For the first time, an individual cell had to be aware of what other cells were doing.
They needed to co-operate with one another. This meant
that whole new chapters of information had to be written
into the DNA code-book, telling cells when they should
grow and when they should not. As soon as such a
mechanism was required, it became possible that it would
go wrong, and the potential for cancer was introduced.

Each cell has between 50,000 and 80,000 genes, each of
which is a small segment of a DNA strand. Every DNA
strand is made up of only four types of molecule, but
these four types of molecule appear over and over again,
in different sequences. Together they form the instructions for producing proteins, which both make up the

fabric of the cell and act as mechanisms regulating its activities. The DNA controls what goes on by making specific kinds of protein, at a particular time, and in particular quantities. Between the genes that produce the proteins that actually carry out these tasks are sequences of DNA that tell those genes when to switch on and off. The role of these regulatory genes is crucial.

There are DNA segments in every normal cell that are involved in growth and development. They produce proteins that allow cells to interact with one another and so permit the healthy functioning of the body and its individual organs. If these genes become disorganised, either through a change in their own genetic code, or through a disruption of the mechanism that controls them, cancer can result. Because of this, they are called oncogenes. Oncogenes perform a function which is very basic to the life of multi-cellular organisms. In evolutionary terms they are extremely old. Something very like a human oncogene is found in fish and flies, and even in yeast.

It was viruses that cause cancer in mice, rats and cats which provided the first clue to the role of oncogenes in the development of tumours. Because these viruses have few genes, it was possible to identify the piece of their DNA that produced a malignant change in cells they infected. To the surprise of the scientists who made the discovery, it became clear that a very similar gene existed in non-cancerous cells from the same animal. Its role was in the control of growth. That is, it was an oncogene. What had happened was that the virus had at some stage picked up this crucial piece of DNA from a cell it infected. The oncogene had then been incorporated into its own genetic structure, and transferred to another cell like a genetic hitch-hiker.

Because certain genes control the activity of others, it is not just the structure of the gene itself that is important, but its position in relation to other genes in the sequence. So the place where the hitch-hiking gene is reinserted is crucial. If it is no longer under the control of its 'minder' gene, it can start to work at an entirely inappropriate time, with disastrous consequences. The same problem can occur if the viral genes insert themselves between a host gene and its on/off switch.

Physically shifting it away from the influences that keep it in check is one way a virus can lead a growth-controlling oncogene to cause cancer. But the concept of genes and their switches also enables us to see how other causes of cancer can work. If the inhibitory gene is altered by a chemical carcinogen or by radiation, for example, the ultimate effect will be the same.

These insights are crucial to our understanding of cancer. Ultimately, this knowledge will also add to our current ability to treat it.

3　Diagnosing Cancer

A variety of symptoms alert us to the fact we may be ill, and persuade us to seek medical advice. In addition to taking note of these symptoms, a doctor checks for further evidence of illness by looking for features that are abnormal, even though they may not have been noticed by the patient. In the case of heart disease, for example, there may be disturbances of heart rhythm that can be heard with a stethoscope, but not otherwise. High blood pressure can sometimes be detected by looking at the blood vessels at the back of the eye. And neurological disease may be reflected in the absence, or unusual strength, of the body's reflexes.

Cancer can begin in almost any organ of the body, and spread to affect any body system. When cancer is suspected, two aspects of diagnosis are borne in mind. The first is definitely to establish whether or not the patient has a tumour, and, if so, to identify the primary site of the disease. The second aspect, which often requires more thorough investigation, is to determine the extent to which the disease has spread. This leads to the concept of 'staging'. A cancer present in one organ, with no evidence of spread, is referred to as Stage I disease. Stage IV cancer, on the other hand, has spread widely around the body. Stages II and III reflect intermediate degrees of spread, but the exact definition differs, depending on the type of tumour.

It is only by mapping the spread of disease in each patient that a suitable plan can be made for treatment. This involves a range of sophisticated tests that provide information on the detailed functioning of any of the organs that may be affected. These include blood and urine tests, X-ray investigations and scans. If there is any suspicion that something is wrong, the physician will arrange for them to be performed. The way these diagnostic tests are carried out may vary from one hospital to another, depending on the equipment and expertise available. But the general principles can be explained. The starting point, though, is to gather information from the patient himself (which is described as 'taking a history') and to conduct a physical examination.

The clinical consultation usually starts with questions about the patient's general well-being, and specific complaints. Particular attention is paid to loss of weight or appetite. A straightforward clinical examination is then performed using well-tried techniques for checking on the state of the chest, heart, abdomen and nervous system. This frequently allows the system of the body that is diseased to be identified. The exact sequence of the examination depends on the symptoms the patient has described. A particular combination of features may suggest a specific diagnosis and a line of investigation that should be followed. Any pallor, which may be due to anaemia, will be noted, and the doctor will feel lymph nodes in the neck, armpits and groin for evidence of enlargement.

Biopsy

The most certain way of diagnosing cancer is to obtain a small sample of the suspect tissue and examine it under the microscope. The tissue obtained is called a biopsy, and the process of examining it, histology. Around 95 per cent of patients with cancer have their disease diagnosed in this way.

Where the tumour is easily accessible (on the skin, for

example), the biopsy can be obtained by making a small incision and removing the abnormal area. It is also straightforward to remove certain lymph nodes suspected of involvement in the disease. But there are many parts of the body that cannot be reached by simple surgery. In these cases, other techniques are used. With the liver, for example, a needle can be passed through the skin and a small core of tissue removed. A similar technique obtains samples from areas within the lungs. If the suspected growth is in the large airways, or bronchi, a fragment of tissue can be snipped out using a small pair of forceps attached to a tube, termed a bronchoscope, which is passed down the windpipe. Similar techniques allow samples to be taken from the stomach and colon.

Whatever the source of the biopsy material, its preparation for histological examination is similar. The tissue is immediately placed in a preserving solution, usually containing formalin, to prevent the growth of bacteria. It is then taken to the laboratory, sliced into thin sections, and stained so that the way the cells are arranged can be clearly seen. The histologist looks for features showing growth has been anarchic and invasive, rather than regular and orderly, as in normal cells.

The cells' shape, appearance, and the way they are dividing often reflect the speed a tumour is growing. So too does the degree of similarity between malignant and healthy cells from the same tissue. Malignancy is not an all-or-nothing change. Taking the intestine as an example, normal, healthy cells develop small projections and secrete mucus. Some malignant cells do the same, although they also have abnormal features. Such cells are said to be well differentiated. Poorly differentiated cells, on the other hand, lose almost all the characteristics of the tissue from which they emerge. Tumours formed from these cells tend to grow more rapidly, and there is a greater risk of spread to the lymph nodes and eventually the liver.

Direct examination of tissue provides so much information about the nature of the disease that biopsy is the cornerstone of cancer diagnosis. But in around 5 per cent of patients, for a variety of reasons, it may not be possible to obtain a sample of the suspect tissue. For example, deep-seated cancers in the pancreas and brain may not be easy to biopsy, especially if a patient is already ill, and unable to tolerate a general anaesthetic. In some circumstances it is still possible to examine suspect cells directly. Samples of sputum and urine may show malignant cells coming from the lung or bladder, for instance.

A final point to be made about biopsy is that the technique is used for the definitive diagnosis of diseases other than cancer. A small sample of tissue from the heart muscle, for example, will provide useful information about the state of the heart; and biopsy of the liver may be crucial to the diagnosis of cirrhosis.

Blood and urine tests

A simple blood sample provides a wealth of information about how the body is working. First of all, there are the blood cells. The number of red and white cells and platelets (cell fragments involved in blood clotting) can be counted electronically. If there are fewer than expected, a disease involving the bone marrow, where such cells are produced, may be the cause. Certain cancers arise in the marrow; some infiltrate it with malignant cells, and others have an indirect effect by secreting substances that suppress its function. It may also be possible to identify malignant changes of the blood cells themselves. This applies mostly to white cells. Red cells and platelets only rarely become malignant.

Much of this information about the state of the blood can now be obtained quickly, automatically, and from very small samples taken from the patient on the ward or in a clinic. One millilitre of blood is placed into a small tube where an anticoagulant chemical prevents it from clotting. In the haematology laboratory, the blood is diluted with a precise amount of saline, and then sucked into a machine which passes a thin stream of blood between two electrodes. The electrodes count the number and size of particles which pass through. It then prints out the count of red cells, white cells and platelets, and a measure of the total amount of haemoglobin (the oxygen-carrying pigment in red cells) which has passed through. Information about the size and shape of cells is also given by the electrical pulses generated each time a cell passes between the electrodes.

When anticoagulated blood is allowed to stand, the red cells start to clump together and settle. The speed with which they do this is called the erythrocyte sedimentation rate, or ESR. This provides another valuable haematological test. In many diseases, including cancer, the ESR is raised because abnormal proteins are present in the blood.

The state of the bone marrow can be assessed by looking at the cells in circulating blood. But it can also be investigated directly by biopsy, in which a sample of marrow is obtained by inserting a fine needle into a cavity inside the sternum, or breast bone. The sternum is rich in marrow, and a small amount can easily be sucked out into a syringe. A larger sample can be obtained from the hip. Where a patient has a cancer (such as one of the lymphomas) which is likely to spread to the bone marrow, such a biopsy is important in staging the disease.

Counting and examining the appearance of blood cells is a useful aid to diagnosis. But biochemical analysis is often also extremely valuable. Blood is an immensely complex mixture of chemicals. Because it bathes cells in every tissue of the body, the blood picks up substances produced by each organ. Levels of these substances can be measured, providing vital evidence about the way an organ is behaving.

The liver, for example, produces a variety of proteins such as serum albumin. When the liver is diseased, perhaps because it is being invaded by a tumour, the blood level of albumin falls, and this can be detected. We can also pick up evidence of liver disease by looking for enzymes that are released when liver cells die, as they will if the organ is being infiltrated by cancer cells. Release of other enzymes also reflects the presence of cancer in bone.

For certain less common tumours there are specific substances that are shed into the blood or urine. Levels of these proteins provide a very accurate reflection of the number of cancer cells present in the body, and so can be used as a precise marker of the growth or shrinking of a cancer. They are therefore an invaluable aid in diagnosis and in monitoring the success of treatment. One of the best examples of tumour markers is found in patients with testicular cancer. In this disease, two proteins are secreted by the tumour, and their level precisely reflects the amount of cancer present.

Other markers include those produced by tumours arising in the endocrine organs, the glands that secrete the body's hormonal messengers. Although these tumours are rare, the markers they produce have been shown to help diagnosis and treatment. It would be valuable to discover similar markers for more common types of cancer, and this is an area where much current research effort is directed. Attempts are also being made to use the antibodies produced by the body's defensive immune system as a guide to the presence of specific types of tumour.

Measuring the levels of particular substances in urine can be as useful as the analysis of blood in providing information about the way organs are working. The concentration of sodium and potassium salts in the urine reflect the health of the kidneys; the presence of bacteria indicates a bladder infection; and certain tumour markers can be found in the urine as well as in the blood. But there are problems in obtaining reliable information from the urine. Unlike the blood, urine can be more or less dilute, depending on the amount of fluid drunk. This means that the concentration of substances it contains differs widely, and it is difficult to distinguish abnormal levels from the background of normal variability. For this reason, most biochemical investigations start with the blood.

X-rays and scans

X-rays can be beamed through the body to produce a photographic image of its internal structures. This is possible because tissues of different density vary in their ability to absorb the radiation. A line drawing of the structures seen on a chest X-ray is shown in figure 3.1. We can see the rib-cage and spine running the length of the X-ray, and the girdle of shoulder bones near the top. In

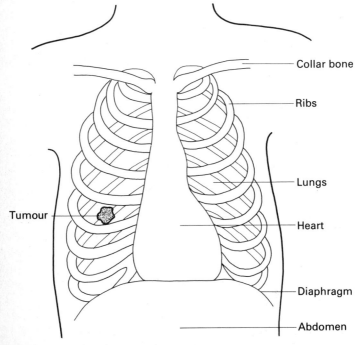

Figure 3.1 Line drawing of the chest showing the features that can be seen in a plain X-ray.

the centre there is a shadow produced by the blood and thick muscle of the heart. The areas of the lungs that are filled with air are not at all dense, and so do not show up well, though small vessels containing blood can be seen.

Straightforward X-rays like this, of the chest, bones and abdomen, provide useful clinical information. A tumour mass in the lung, for example, is more dense than the surrounding air-filled tissue, and shows up as a shadow. If the mass compresses one of the bronchi, air may be prevented from reaching a large part of the lung, and the opaque area will be substantial. In these circumstances, X-rays can show there is something that needs further investigation, though they do not tell us whether the mass is benign or malignant. 'Plain' X-rays are also very useful in locating the site of metastases in bone, when someone is already known to have cancer. Areas that have been invaded by tumour cells show up as blemishes, which may be either lighter or darker than the surrounding healthy bone.

But plain X-rays are limited. Where different kinds of tissue absorb radiation to the same extent, it is impossible to distinguish between them. For example, if a primary cancer of the colon produces secondary tumours in the liver, they cannot usually be detected by a plain X-ray of the abdomen. Similarly, an X-ray of the skull does not reveal enough information about the brain to allow tumours there to be detected. A bullet lodged within the skull can be seen, but the density of a tumour is so similar to that of normal tissue that there is no difference in appearance on an ordinary X-ray film.

Some of these problems can be overcome by using 'contrast' techniques. The simplest example is the barium meal. The patient swallows a fluid containing barium sulphate (which is harmless, rapidly excreted, and not absorbed in the intestine). The fluid blocks X-rays, and the areas it occupies show up white on an X-ray film. Swallowing barium allows the lining of the oesophagus, stomach and small intestine to be seen clearly, and any abnormality picked out. Barium can also be inserted into the rectum, so that the colon is visualised. Sometimes both barium and air are used – the 'double contrast' enema. Here, the colon fills up with air and barium tracks around the inner walls, highlighting any defects. Blockages can easily be seen since the barium does not track beyond them, or does so only slowly.

Such contrast studies give a clear indication of the site of the problem, and often provide good evidence of whether the growth is benign or malignant. Characteristically, a cancer has pronounced edges and a raised centre. Benign ulcers tend to be flat and shallow, without raised edges.

Another major type of contrast study involves injecting into the blood a dye that blocks X-rays. The radio-opaque dye circulates around the body, eventually becoming concentrated in the kidneys. There it passes through the tiny collecting tubes within the kidney and then, via the ureter, into the bladder. Shortly after injection, the kidneys, ureters and bladder should all be clearly outlined on an X-ray photograph. The technique, known as an intravenous urogram (or IVU), reveals the site of any blockages and shows whether lymph nodes, which may have become enlarged with metastases, are increasing pressure on the ureters at the back of the abdomen.

It is also possible to study individual veins and arteries using contrast media. After injection through a small needle, X-rays allow the radio- opaque dye to be followed through the blood vessels, revealing blockages and any sites where pressure from a primary tumour or metastasis has caused the vein or artery to deviate from its normal course.

Contrast media increase the value of X-rays for diagnosis. But the most revolutionary advance of the past 20 years has been the invention of Computerised Tomography (or CT scanning). The English physicist Geoffrey Hounsfield first described the technique in 1972, and was awarded a Nobel prize four years later. By linking X-ray machines to sophisticated computers, it is now possible to obtain clear images that reveal very small differences between types of tissue.

The principle behind the technique is simple. Instead of having one source of X-rays, and one photographic plate, a whole battery of X-ray sources and detectors is moved around the patient. The body is 'looked at' from every angle, and a single image built up on a computer by pooling the information obtained. This image reflects the

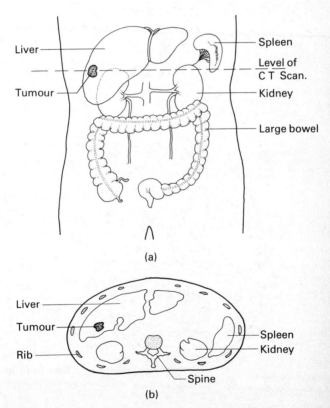

(a)

(b)

Figure 3.2 (a) Anatomical features of the abdomen showing a tumour in the liver (b) The features shown in (a) as they appear on a CT scan through the abdomen.

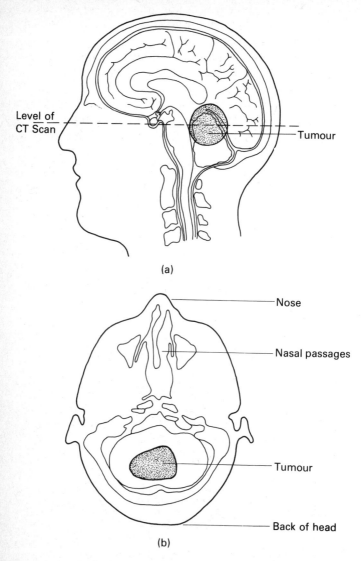

Level of CT Scan

Tumour

(a)

Nose

Nasal passages

Tumour

Back of head

(b)

Figure 3.3 (a) A cross-section of the anatomy of the head showing the position of a tumour (b) Details evident on a CT scan, showing the precise location of a brain tumour.

precise density of the tissue at thousands of different points within the body. It can also be used very effectively to reveal structures within the skull. One remarkable feature of the CT image is that it represents not a straight-forward view from the front, back or side, but a cross-section through the patient. (See figures 3.2 and 3.3.)

By moving the machine along the length of the body, a series of cross-sections can be obtained – almost as if the patient were in an optical bacon slicer. In this way, information is available about the depth of a tumour, as well as its length and breadth, and its precise position within the body. This third dimension allows the total volume of a tumour to be calculated. The X-rays used in radiotherapy can be directed more precisely, so that the tumour is 'hit', and surrounding healthy tissue spared. And the shrinking of a tumour with therapy can be accurately assessed.

CT scanners are expensive. They cost around £250,000 to buy and install, and nearly as much again each year to run. The information they reveal is much the same as could be obtained using other techniques, but the other methods are often more lengthy, complicated, and un-pleasant. CT scanners therefore save time and discom-fort. Most large hospitals should now have a CT scanner, and all patients have access to them.

Nuclear Magnetic Resonance (NMR) scanning is a still more recent technique. It is also yet more expensive: NMR scanners cost around £1 million. The device does not use X-rays. Instead, the body is placed in an enor-mously strong magnetic field. Nuclei within the atoms (that ultimately make up cells and tissue) align themselves in a particular direction, like tiny bar magnets. The patient is then exposed to a brief pulse from a radio-frequency beam. This throws the nuclei out of alignment, and as they spin back they themselves emit signals at different frequencies, like small radio transmitters.

The nuclei that make up different chemical elements emit different sorts of signal. The concentration of an element varies according to the tissue present, and plotting the sources of the various kinds of signal produces an image of the internal structures of the body. At the moment, the images available from NMR scanners are as good as those produced by computerised tomography. But the ultimate advantage of NMR may well lie in the fact that it gives information not just about the location of different tissues, but also about the biochemical processes going on inside them.

NMR is already being used to plot the changes that occur in heart muscle when it is deprived of oxygen. Similar techniques will be able to reveal what is going on inside tumours that are exposed to radiation or drugs. This will increase our understanding of cancer and how to treat it, and it is probably in a research capacity that NMR will be most valuable to oncology. But we will also see increasing use of NMR scanners for diagnosis. Though the idea of strong magnetic fields and radio beams may seem dangerous, NMR will probably prove more safe than techniques based on X-rays, which themselves carry only a very low risk of causing damage.

There are two other types of scan. The first is ultrasound. This technique employs high frequency sound waves, as used in underwater sonar. The energy waves penetrate the body and bounce back, producing an image. Echoes come back particularly strongly from areas where there is a change in the density of tissue: for example, around a fluid-filled tumour. Ultrasound images are more difficult to interpret than CT scans. But the technique is easy, safe, relatively cheap, and in expert hands can provide valuable diagnostic information.

Radioisotope scans are different again. The patient takes a radioactive substance, which becomes incorporated into tissue. Its distribution can then be mapped using a camera sensitive to the radiation emitted. Bone scanning provides a good example.

Healthy bone is always taking up phosphate, which is one of its main constituents. The patient is given an intravenous injection of phosphate that has been labelled with a radioactive tracer. Time is allowed for the phosphate to circulate around the body, and for it to be taken up by bone cells. A radioactivity detector is then placed in front of the patient. Where the uptake of phosphate is greater, as it will be if tumour cells are present (and also, for example, if there is arthritis or a bone infection), 'hotspots' of radioactivity can be seen on the image produced of the body. The information given by the isotope scan can be checked with evidence from X-rays, and from the patient's own reports about bone pain, and appropriate treatment planned.

Radioactive isotopes are also widely used when there is a tumour in the brain or liver. Normally, large molecules in the blood are prevented from entering brain tissue. But this barrier breaks down where there is a tumour, and a suitable molecule labelled with a radioactive isotope can show where this leakage occurs. In the case of the liver, the labelled isotope cannot enter areas where there is tumour, and the position of the disease is shown on the scan by the absence of radioactivity.

Existing scanning techniques are always being improved, and new ones developed. Together with the range of tests that tell us how well various organs in the body are functioning, they help build up a complete picture of the disease. This information is vital if cancer and its symptoms are to be treated effectively.

4 Surgery

Surgery is probably the oldest branch of medicine. Since prehistory, man has known that certain diseases can be effectively treated by removing the affected organ. So there are many centuries of experience contributing to our understanding of surgical techniques and how they should be applied. The patient with cancer meets the surgeon for one (or more) of three reasons: to diagnose the disease, to treat it, and to control its symptoms.

The first use of surgery is in establishing the exact nature of the disease by taking samples of the tumour for detailed investigation. Obtaining the tissue specimen is called biopsy, and its examination under a microscope is histology. Following the original biopsy, the surgeon may also take samples from organs or tissues at some distance from the original site of the cancer. This is to check whether the disease has spread.

Secondly, the surgeon may be involved in the attempt to cure the tumour by its removal. Surgery on its own may be sufficient to deal with up to 40 per cent of all malignant tumours. But it is important to realise that the decision to treat a particular cancer by surgery says nothing about the severity of the disease. We now understand fairly well which types of tumour are best tackled by surgery, and which by other forms of treatment. Many tumours are equally well, and perhaps better, treated by radiation or chemotherapy. So patients who learn that their disease is not to be treated by surgery should not be depressed. 'Inoperable' says nothing about the curability of a particular cancer.

The third reason for surgery is to help control symptoms. This may mean an operation to bypass obstructions to the normal passage of food in the bowel, for example, or to sever nerves that carry the sensation of pain from a part of the body to the brain. The latter technique is particularly helpful in relieving pain without using heavy doses of drugs.

Surgery as an aid to diagnosis

Most patients first notice something wrong when they discover a lump, or loss of blood, or feel pain. Usually, the sign that first arouses suspicion is a lump, in the breast or neck, for example. After the patient has seen a general practitioner, and simple explanations for the swelling have been considered and discounted, the patient is referred to a surgeon.

Often there is an obvious cause, such as an infection, which can be easily dealt with. But if the surgeon is in any doubt at all about the nature of the swelling he will nearly always recommend removal of the lump or a specimen from it for investigation in the laboratory. The purpose is to see whether the cells that make up the specimen show the orderly features of normal growth, or the disorganised appearance of cancer. Examination is by powerful microscope, with the aid of chemical stains which allow different parts of the cell to be clearly seen.

The role of biopsy is illustrated by breast cancer. Although the great majority of breast lumps (roughly nine out of ten) are completely innocent, it is impossible to tell which are not without taking a specimen for examination. The prospect even of minor surgery, such as breast biopsy, naturally causes anxiety. But a biopsy is recommended so that the doctor can be sure there is no serious problem. This cautious, 'better safe than sorry' approach is in the best interests of the patient; and it is worth the slight discomfort to exclude the possibility of malignant disease or, where cancer is found, to start treatment early.

The extent of a breast biopsy depends on the site, size and nature of the lump. Many breast lumps can have fluid drawn from their interior by means of a needle no larger than the one used to take blood samples from a vein. The fluid contains sufficient cells for a diagnosis to be made. With more solid lumps a small core of tissue, like a thin strand of spaghetti, can be removed using a slightly larger hollow needle. This operation is carried out under local anaesthetic: a chemical which temporarily stops the transmission of nerve impulses to the brain is injected into the skin, making the procedure completely painless.

Larger lumps may require what is known as an open biopsy. An incision is made in the skin above the lump, and the swelling removed. This can be done under local anaesthetic, but many surgeons prefer a general anaesthetic for this more extensive kind of biopsy.

Before any kind of operation, under either local or general anaesthetic, patients are asked to sign a form confirming they understand what the procedure involves and that they consent to it. This is not a formality. It should be taken as seriously by the patient as it is by the surgeon. In some cases a further point arises. If biopsy shows that cancer is present, it may be in the patient's best interest to remove the whole tumour immediately. This saves the patient undergoing another operation, and reduces the risk the cancer will spread. So people are sometimes asked to consent not only to the exploratory operation but also to any further surgery that may be judged necessary.

People often fear that having given consent to a small, routine biopsy, they may wake to find that a much more serious operation has been performed. In the case of a breast lump, for example, the anxiety may be that the whole breast will be removed. Another common fear is that a patient undergoing an exploratory operation for suspected bowel cancer will wake to find a colostomy (in which the bowel is opened out onto the wall of the abdomen) has been fashioned without their approval.

Any patient worried that something like this may happen should explain their fears to the doctor, and ask specifically if any of these more extensive procedures is being contemplated. All patients are entitled to refuse permission for the surgeon to proceed to any further form of treatment. It may be that they want more time to think about the operation; perhaps the desire is to obtain a second opinion. Though the surgeon always has the well-being of the patient uppermost in his mind, it is vital that no-one feels they have been forced to undergo a procedure to which they did not fully agree. It is far better that any fears are expressed before the operation than that a misunderstanding should lead to anger and resentment later.

In a few cases, the surgeon will already be reasonably confident he knows the nature of the lump he is about to biopsy. He may then specifically request consent to proceed to a more substantial operation if the diagnosis is confirmed. In the case of a breast lump, the tumour can be removed and sent to the pathology laboratory where it is quickly frozen and cross-sections taken for immediate examination. The patient is still anaesthetised in the operating theatre. If cancer is diagnosed, the surgeon can then extend the area of tissue cut out, and, if necessary, remove the breast – provided that surgeon and patient have agreed in advance that this would be the best course.

Staging cancer

We have already considered the concept of staging: outlining the extent of spread of a tumour at the time it makes its first symptoms felt. This is really a part of diagnosis. In certain kinds of cancer, staging is vital in determining treatment. One example is the lymphomas, a group of cancers of the lymphatic system which may affect any lymph gland in the body. Here, the extent of disease decides whether the patient is treated with radiation, or chemotherapy, or both.

Even sophisticated modern diagnostic equipment, such as CT scanning, cannot always provide the information the oncologist requires. When this happens, surgery can have a role to play. In the case of a lymphoma, the surgeon may be asked to open the patient's abdomen (an operation called laparotomy) to inspect and remove certain of the lymph glands that lie at the back of the abdominal cavity. In expert hands, a laparotomy is a safe and simple procedure and means that the patient receives the treatment that is most appropriate for his or her particular case. The exact circumstances under which laparotomy is necessary are considered later.

Cancer surgery

Surgery acquired scientific foundations around the turn of the last century. It became clear then that surgeons sometimes failed to cure their patients because cancer had spread to form secondary tumours away from the original site of disease. Removal of the primary cancer alone – however expertly it was done, and even if the whole of the affected organ, such as the stomach or breast was cut out – was not sufficient to save life if the patient later went on to develop disease at some distant site. This new understanding of the biology of tumours was a turning point in the treatment of malignant disease. From it came the realisation that surgery had to pay attention to the paths along which tumours tend to spread. The result was an approach termed 'radical' surgery, in which the technique is to remove both the affected organ and the surrounding lymph nodes, preferably all in one piece.

The mastectomy operation originated by the American surgeon William Halsted, which involved removal of the complete breast and the lymph nodes stretching right up into the armpit, was one of the first examples. Similar techniques to remove the uterus, ovaries, fallopian tubes and lymph nodes in the pelvis, were developed by Wertheim in Vienna as a way of treating gynaecological cancer. A skin tumour on the back of the hand came to be treated not just by removal of the cancer itself and the area immediately surrounding it, but by excision of all the skin within five centimetres of the tumour's edge. In some cases, lymph nodes in the armpit were also removed.

Techniques of extended, radical surgery undoubtedly improved the chances a patient would survive the malignant disease. But the drawback was that such extensive procedures were more difficult for the patient to withstand, and the incidence of side-effects, even from expert surgery, became considerable. Nevertheless, radical surgery remained the mainstay of cancer therapy for many years.

Fortunately, recent developments in many spheres of medicine mean that radical cancer surgery can be more effective than ever, whilst at the same time its safety is increased. Improved surgical and anaesthetic techniques allow extensive operations with far fewer side-effects. When Halsted first described his operation, anaesthesia consisted of chloroform dabbed on a piece of cloth held over the patient's face. Now there is an immense variety of anaesthetic agents, which can be precisely administered, and their effects monitored. Blood transfusion is universally available as a way of counteracting collapse of the circulation, which used to be a common and dangerous feature of major surgery. And serious post-operative infections are now extremely rare, thanks to sterile operating conditions and the judicious use of antibiotics.

The preparation of patients for surgery is also much more thorough. People with other medical conditions, such as chronic bronchitis, can be brought into hospital for treatment, often weeks prior to surgery, to make them as fit as possible to withstand the operation. And techniques which allow a patient to be fed through a drip line inserted into a vein ensure that people who have been unwell and losing weight can be 'built up' before surgery.

At the same time, advances in radiation and drug treatment are supplementing the good that can be done by the surgeon's knife. The concept of treating not only the primary tumour but also its paths of spread, learned from the pioneer surgeons, can be applied also in radiotherapy. This means that a less extensive operation is complemented by radiation directed at sites to which the tumour may have spread. In place of Halsted's radical mastectomy, which is now only rarely performed, we have a conservative 'simple' mastectomy followed by radiation treatment of the adjacent lymph glands. This can destroy tumour left behind at surgery as effectively as if the glands had been physically removed during the operation; and the patient benefits from surgery which is less disfiguring and easier to recover from. Also, the chances of side-effects, such as a permanently swollen arm, are now much less.

In bowel cancer, too, radiotherapy has combined with surgery to improve the effectiveness of treatment. Many colon cancers grow into local structures, such as the muscles of the abdominal wall, sometimes making it technically impossible for the surgeon to remove the tumour. Radiation prior to the operation can so shrink the tumour that surgery once again becomes feasible.

Both these examples show that the management of cancer has become a collaborative effort. In very few cases will a patient be treated by a single specialist. To exploit the maximum advantage from recent progress in the treatment of malignant disease, a combination of approaches is often required.

But there are some patients who will benefit only from very major surgery, and it is clear that such procedures will cause anxiety. It may be helpful to remember that however simple or serious the surgery, there is no time in the patient's life when more people will be concentrating on his well-being than during the two or three hours he spends in the operating theatre. If we count the people involved in nursing, anaesthetic and surgical care, it is common to find between 20 and 30 specialists there for the single purpose of ensuring that a particular patient receives the highest possible standards of treatment.

Surgical treatment of symptoms

Apart from its role in the diagnosis, staging and treatment of cancer, surgery can be used to alleviate many of the symptoms caused by the disease. Despite recent advances, there are patients who cannot be cured. But this does not mean we are powerless to prolong life and relieve distress. Knowing the natural development of cancer allows us to anticipate events, and be ready with help when problems occur.

There are many examples of what can be done. For example, certain tumours which grow in the oesophagus, or gullet, may eventually block the passage of food and even liquid. If this happens, a rigid metal or plastic tube can be inserted into the oesophagus to restore an opening and so allow food to pass through. Though this treatment is not itself aimed at tackling the tumour, it may allow the patient's strength to recover to a point where further surgery is possible, or provide time for a course of radiotherapy to be given.

Occasionally problems arise because of the treatment rather than the disease. Where radiotherapy of oesophageal cancer is successful, the radiation itself occasionally causes tight bands to form around the muscular tube, making it difficult to swallow solid food. The surgeon may be able to pass rods of increasingly large diameter down the oesophagus, gradually dilating it and so restoring normal swallowing.

Both these techniques are useful in helping patients with oesophageal cancer, but 'internal rearrangements' can be made to bypass the effects of many other diseases.

Bladder cancer provides an example. Tumours that block the flow of urine into or out of the bladder can cause pressure to build up in the kidneys, and lead eventually to kidney failure if untreated. However, it is relatively simple to divert the urinary passages away from the bladder, and even to make an artificial reservoir out of a piece of the patient's intestine. Urine can then be made to flow freely through a hole made in the skin, into an appropriate container.

But perhaps the most dramatic contribution that surgery can make to the relief of symptoms is in the control of pain. Pain sensations are transmitted to the brain along special fibres contained in the nerves. When these fibres reach the spinal cord, they occupy a particular place on the edge of the spinal column, forming two pathways, one on each side of the body. When pain is a severe problem, it is sometimes possible to block these pathways, and so prevent pain impulses passing from the affected part of the body to the brain. This can be achieved by injecting an anaesthetic drug into the nerve itself, or by actually destroying the pathway in the spinal cord at the level of the neck.

Many hospitals have created special clinics for the treatment of pain caused by a range of diseases, including cancer. In expert hands, the procedures outlined are safe, can be carried out with the patient awake using only local anaesthetic, and bring instantaneous and complete pain relief. Awareness that pain can be helped by methods other than massive doses of drugs is spreading.

Reconstructive surgery

Helping restore the normal appearance of the body after successful removal of a tumour is another role for surgery. The most well-known example is probably breast reconstruction after mastectomy. Though accepting that it often forms part of the best treatment available, many women understandably feel disfigured by the loss of a breast.

After a period of observation to ensure there is no recurrence of the tumour, the surgeon many find it possible, in some patients, to reconstruct the breast. This involves another operation in which an incision is made in the skin and an artificial breast-shaped implant, or prosthesis, inserted to recreate a normal shape. Though not suitable in all cases, there is no doubt this form of cosmetic surgery is a valuable step along the road to psychological, as well as physical, recovery from cancer.

Reconstructive surgery has advanced enormously over the past few years. With the aid of skin grafts and microscopic surgery, it is now possible to refashion whole areas of anatomy that have been removed to treat a tumour. The most striking examples are found in patients who have had their jaws and faces 'remade' after excision of cancers of the mouth, tongue and the sinus of the cheek bone.

There is little doubt that some patients delay seeking medical advice for what they believe to be cancer because they fear the consequences of extensive surgery. If knowledge of modern reconstructive techniques were more widely available, it is possible more patients would go to their doctors at an earlier stage, and so improve their chances of successful treatment.

Transplantation

Transplant surgery generates interest and emotion, and it may have a small part to play in the treatment of cancer. Although still largely used for non-malignant conditions, such as degeneration of the heart muscle and kidney failure, there are a few instances in which cancer patients can be helped. The best example is that of primary tumour of the liver.

If cancer is confined to the liver, removal of the tumour

is likely to cure the patient. But no-one can survive unless they have a substantial amount of functioning liver. This means that patients with large tumours cannot have them removed. Even if the cancer were eradicated, the patient would still die. Advances in transplanation mean that it is now possible to remove completely the diseased liver from the cancer patient, and replace it with a healthy organ obained from a human donor. Experience with this form of treatment is growing rapidly, and results are increasingly good.

But for cancer as a whole, transplantation has little to offer. By the time the disease has reached the point where the whole organ needs removal, cancer has usually spread to distant parts of the body.

'Second look' operations

Despite recent advances in diagnosis, there are still times following treatment when the only way to check up on a patient's progess is to operate and look at the affected part of the body. This may be done even though the patient has no signs or symptoms of disease and feels perfectly well. There are two reasons for this kind of surgical investigation. If the operation shows no evidence of cancer, the patient can be reassured that everything is well. If there is cancer present, it is likely that the amount of tumour is small and that it will therefore respond more completely to treatment than if it had been left to grow until symptoms appeared.

In patients who have had part of their intestines re-moved for cancer of the bowel, followed by radiation treatment or chemotherapy, it is relatively common for a 'second look' laparotomy to be performed. This also hap-pens after treatment for cancer of the ovaries. And there is no doubt that patients' lives have sometimes been saved by such check-up operations. Like everything else in medicine, the value of such surgery is constantly under review, and more sophisticated techniques of imaging the body, or means of detecting tumours by finding markers in the blood, may come to replace it.

Summary

In summary, surgery is invaluable in the diagnosis and treatment of cancer, and in palliating its effects. But rather than being our only effective treatment for cancer, it now takes its place alongside other successful approaches to the disease, and is often used in conjunction with them. Surgery is now safer and far more skilled and precise than it used to be. Surgical procedures for tackling cancer are often less damaging, and fear of an operation should never cause a patient to delay seeking proper medical advice.

5 Radiotherapy

Discovery, and early success

The use of radiation to treat disease must often seem a mysterious process. Though the machinery responsible is in evidence, the delivery of radiation itself cannot be seen. Also we associate radiation – whether from nuclear weapons or the risk from power stations – with causing disease rather than curing it. So it is worth explaining what radiation is, how its medically useful forms are produced, and how its beneficial effects occur.

Radiation is the spreading out of energy from a point. The ripples in a pond that follow the throwing in of a stone are one example of radiated energy: the sound waves that enable you to hear the splash are another. So too is radiated heat, such as we receive from the sun, or from a household 'radiator'. Light is radiating energy, as are radio and television signals. These last three forms, known as electromagnetic radiation, differ from sound waves in that they can travel through empty space.

Just as with ripples on a pond, electromagnetic radiation has a 'wavelength' – the distance between the top of one wave to the top of the next. Radiowaves and radar are at the long-wavelength end of the electromagnetic spectrum. The waves that form visible light are of intermediate length; and the radiation used in therapy is of short wavelength. (Figure 5.1 shows their position in the spectrum.) The two major forms of radiation employed in

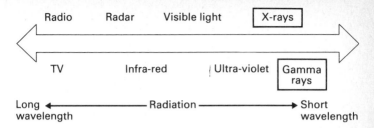

Figure 5.1 The electromagnetic spectrum. Radiation used in cancer treatment is at the short-wavelength end.

radiotherapy are X-rays and gamma rays. Unlike visible light, both penetrate body tissues.

In the case of X-rays, this property is put to good use as an aid to diagnosis. X-rays pass easily through soft tissue, such as skin and muscle, but are blocked by bone. This means that if a photographic plate sensitive to the rays is placed behind part of the patient's body, an image of the internal structures can be obtained. Exposure to the X-rays used in diagnosis has to be carefully monitored because excessive amounts damage tissue – and that is an unwelcome side-effect. But putting this destructive power to controlled use is the essence of radiotherapy.

We owe the discovery of X-rays (in 1895) to the German physicist, Wilhelm Konrad Roentgen. As with many scientific advances, the discovery was an accident. Roentgen was investigating the properties of electrons (which are negatively-charged subatomic particles) when he discovered that rays capable of blackening photographic film were being produced. Since they had never before been noticed, he called them X-rays – the 'X' standing for 'unknown'.

The first apparatus for reliably producing these rays was invented a few years later by an American, Dr Coolidge. His invention, the Coolidge tube, remains the basis of modern equipment for generating X-rays. A beam of electrons is produced by a heated metal filament and directed towards a metal plate. When the electrons hit the plate, part of the energy of movement which they lose is converted into X-rays, which shoot away at great speed. The amount of energy which the X-rays carry depends on the force with which the electron beam has impacted on the metal plate, and can be varied. High-energy X-rays penetrate further into body tissue than low-energy ones.

Within a few years of their discovery, X-rays were being used in treatment. Surprisingly, considering the number of factors involved in the selection of patients, this early therapy was extremely successful. It was fortunate that patients with tumours on the surface of the skin were among the first to be treated. The low-energy X-rays available at the time would not have had much impact on deep-seated tumours, but were sufficiently powerful to produce dramatic improvements in superficial cancers. And because these tumours were easily visible, the success of treatment was immediately apparent. Heartened by these early cures, doctors used radiation treatment of one form or another against a wide range of diseases. Among conditions frequently treated by radiation in the early years of this century were tuberculosis (or TB), peptic ulcers, chronic ear infections, and the skin diseases ring worm, scabies and eczema. The one thing these diseases had in common was that they were untreatable by any other method at the time.

The success radiation achieved with these diseases was wider than is often realised. But the most spectacular results were obtained in the treatment of cancer. Radiation, used either alone or with surgery, saved the lives of many patients. Where cure was not possible, intractable symptoms such as bone pain and the ulceration and bleeding caused by tumours were relieved. All this happened at a time when the only alternative was morphine or brandy.

From the very beginning of radiotherapy, there were two, complementary approaches. One was the delivery of radiation in the form of X-rays directed at the patient from a device containing an X-ray tube. This treatment from a radiation source outside the patient is known as teletherapy ('tele' meaning 'at a distance'). But there is also a form of treatment in which the source of radioactivity is placed inside the patient. This is especially effective in tackling cancers that arise within a body cavity, such as the mouth or uterus.

The technique is to implant radioactive needles or 'seeds' within the diseased tissue, or to place alongside it a container with a radioactive source inside. This form of therapy relies on materials which emit radiation spontaneously as they decay. The realisation that such materials existed was as important to medicine and physics as the discovery of X-rays. At much the same time as Roentgen was making his momentous observation, Marie Curie, in Paris, was working to extract the first tenth of a gram of a naturally-occurring radioactive element (later known as radium) from tons of pitchblende ore. She succeeded in 1898. This element emits gamma radiation, which is identical to X-rays, except for the way it is produced.

Radium was the first element identified as a source of radiation. But it has now largely been replaced by artificial sources based on caesium and cobalt. These are radioactive forms (called isotopes) of natural elements, created by placing the original material in an atomic reactor.

The clinical use of implanted radioactive sources was as quick to develop as the medical application of X-rays. It was found particularly effective in the treatment of gynaecological cancers. Progress in both forms of radiotherapy was due partly to trial and error, and partly to the discovery of new sources of radiation, and more sophisticated techniques for delivering it to the patient. But it also depended on increased understanding of the effects radiation has on living tissue – a branch of science known as radiobiology – and on our expanding knowledge about radiation itself. It became clear from discoveries in physics that X-rays fitted into the spectrum of electromagnetic radiation we have already seen in figure 5.1. It was also apparent that the effect of a particular form of radiation depends on its wavelength: as the wavelength becomes shorter, the energy it contains increases. Ultraviolet light near the visible spectrum is of relatively long wavelength. It produces suntan after a summer's day spent on the beach. But a few minutes' exposure to powerful X-ray machines, delivering high-intensity short-wavelength radiation can cause marked reddening and soreness of the skin.

Early pioneers of radiation thought that X-rays were harmless, and frequently exposed themselves unnecessarily by placing a hand in the radiation beam to see if the X-ray tube had 'warmed up'. When they could see an image of their finger bones cast on the wall, they knew the machine was ready for use. It was not then appreciated that bombardment by X-rays affects all living tissues and that radiation can have very long-term as well as immediate effects. In fact, casual attitudes to the use of X-rays persisted into the 1950s, when High Street shoe shops had X-ray machines to establish whether or not shoes fitted. This was a clear case of people being needlessly exposed to radiation.

Even in the earliest days of X-rays, it was realised that tissues which divided and grew rapidly were the most obviously affected by radiation. It had been learned that a patient whose scalp was irradiated lost his hair, and that irradiation of the abdomen caused diarrhoea because the fast-growing cells lining the gut were destroyed. But the same amount of radiation, received from the same beam, was recognised to have no noticeable effect on tissues such as the skull or spine.

Principles underlying treatment

The science of radiobiology has been long unfolding. But we can now use what we know about radiation and its effects to plan treatment so that maximum damage is done to the tumour, and as little as possible to healthy tissue. The following points summarise our understanding, and how it is applied to ensure effective and safe treatment.

1   All tissues are affected by radiation. The more frequently a tissue's cells divide, the more quickly the effects are seen. But slowly dividing tissues are just as profoundly affected by radiation, though it may take many years for the effects to become apparent. This means that treatment should be confined as closely as possible to the tissues that contain the malignant cells.

2   If they are well nourished, cancer cells are slightly more susceptible to radiation than their healthy counterparts. Radiation can therefore be used to destroy cancer without affecting healthy tissue so severely.

3   Although well-nourished cancer cells are sensitive to radiation, not all cancer cells are well nourished. Some cells, particularly those at the centre of tumours, are poorly supplied with blood and so lack oxygen. This makes the cells resistant to the effects of radiation. We therefore expect radiation to work best in relatively small tumours where each cell is well supplied with oxygen.

4   Radiation is more successful against a tumour if it is given in several small amounts over a period of weeks rather than as a single dose. This is because the well-nourished cancer cells on the outside of the tumour are destroyed by the first bombardment of radiation. More oxygen and nutrients then diffuse into the tumour, enriching cells that were previously deficient, and so making them more sensitive to the doses of radiation that follow. This is the reason most courses of radiation are arranged over several weeks – in which case the dose is said to be 'fractionated'.

5   Irradiating different parts of the body has different side-effects. Nausea and vomiting are more pronounced when radiation is directed towards the

middle of the body. Large amounts of radiation can be delivered to extremities such as the hands and feet without noticeable effect. Yet a small dose applied to the 'solar plexus' can make patients feel unwell.

Radiotherapists use this knowledge to judge how much radiation should be given at each session to each patient, taking into account the area of the body that needs to be treated. Combined with experience of the total amount of radiation needed to kill the tumour, the exact number of treatments required in a particular course can be calculated. The large number of factors that have to be taken into account is the reason that each course of radiation treatment is different. In good practice, there is no such thing as a 'standard' course of radiotherapy. Every patient is unique. The size of their tumours varies; so does their individual response to radiation. There may even be geographical differences.

When radiotherapy is the best treatment

Many factors are considered when deciding whether a particular patient can be helped by radiation. Although some people are still disappointed to find their disease is 'inoperable', this is by no means always a disadvantage. Radiation cannot be directly compared with surgery. Some cancers are best treated by surgical removal. Others are better tackled by radiation. The two approaches are complementary and not competitive attempts at dealing with cancer.

Surgery is excellent for tumours which arise in a part of the body which can be removed without causing too much damage. One example of this would be cancer involving a portion of the bowel. But cancers often develop in surgically inaccessible places, such as deep within the brain. We also know that for many tumours removal of the primary cancer alone will not be adequate treatment. Total eradication means removal not only of the initial tumour but also of the many sites to which it may have spread. The area of tissue that would need to be cut out could be unacceptably large, and in these cases surgery may be as dangerous as the disease itself.

On the other hand, certain tumours are found in tissues which are just as sensitive to radiation as the cancer itself, and perhaps even more sensitive. The lens of the eye provides a good example. Even small doses of radiation risk the formation of cataracts. Where radiation may cause as many problems as it solves, surgery is often preferred.

Surgery and radiotherapy have in common the fact that they are local treatments: they deal with cancer in a particular area of the body. With surgery, this is clear. Cutting out a cancer in the bowel is an effective way of removing the primary tumour, but will obviously not deal with a secondary cancer that might have developed in the lung. In a similar way, radiation can be very effective in the places where it is directed, but will have no effect on disease in distant parts of the body. Because these secondary areas of cancer may cause symptoms and threaten life, cancer is often best considered a 'systemic' disease; that is, one that affects the whole body. Cancers that have spread may therefore need systemic treatment, such as with drugs. The difference between local and systemic disease, each with their appropriate treatments, is another example of the way choice of therapy has to be tailored to meet the needs of the individual patient.

Although many people feel 'cheated' if their condition cannot be treated by an operation, there are many circumstances in which radiotherapy is just as effective, and often much less troublesome to the patient. One example is cancer of the prostate, where tumours can often be perfectly well controlled by radiation alone. Treatment usually takes between four and six weeks, with the patient based at home, though travelling to hospital several times a week for sessions of radiotherapy. Because radiation is directed towards the pelvis, which contains the bladder and many feet of bowel, there may be temporary discomfort passing urine, and some diarrhoea. But the chance of cure is good, and if treatment is successful the patient is left with a perfectly normal bladder and bowel. There is no problem of incontinence, and urine can be passed in the usual way. Sexual function is also unaffected.

In contrast, radical surgery for prostate cancer is designed to remove the gland itself and much of the tissue that surrounds it. Such extensive surgery produces an equally good chance of cure, but may mean that a patient becomes incontinent and has to wear some form of protective clothing for the rest of his life. In a small number of cases, he will also become impotent because of treatment.

Side-effects of radiotherapy

Radiotherapy is surrounded by myths. In the early days of treatment, when equipment was primitive and our understanding of radiation poor, many severe side-effects were found. Memories from these days have been perpetuated; but the position is quite different today. Most patients believe radiation will cause hair to fall out, produce severe burns, intense nausea and vomiting, and leave people permanently weak. So they are often pleasantly surprised to reach the end of a course of treatment without any of these side-effects occurring. That this misunderstanding about radiation is still so widespread shows communication between doctors and patients can be improved. Any type of treatment involves a balance between desired and disadvantageous effects. But with modern equipment and practice, there is no reason to think the balance will be anything but positive.

One of the problems that faces doctor and patient alike is that too little is said about cancer. Because of this it is easy for the effects of treatment to become confused with the effects of the disease itself. If, for example, a patient with advanced lung cancer develops a painful secondary tumour somewhere in the bone, the patient will quite rightly be offered radiotherapy to reduce the discomfort. This treatment is given to help with a symptom, and it is not expected that the patient will live any longer because of it.

In some cases, the patient will receive radiation and then die shortly afterwards from the effects of his advanced disease. If the reason for the treatment was not fully understood, and the patient's condition not properly appreciated, his family and friends may date his decline from the time treatment was started. His death may even be blamed on the radiotherapy, when in fact it was due simply to the progress of the disease. It is often easier to think that the treatment caused the deterioration, and not the disease. To accept that the person died because he smoked cigarettes, which caused him to get lung cancer, sometimes brings the unspeakable threat too close to home. This example is only one of the ways in which myths about treatment can develop.

What happens in radiotherapy?

Many important decisions are taken before a patient reaches a radiotherapy department. Once the disease has been diagnosed, various tests (described in chapter 3) reveal the kind of cancer that is involved and how far it has spread. The patient's individual circumstances and symptoms are considered, and only then is a decision made about the best form of treatment.

Let us assume that a patient has a form of cancer that is most usefully treated by radiation alone. To make the example more precise, take as an illustration a young woman with cancer of the cervix, or neck of the womb. She is likely to have gone to her GP because of bleeding or discharge from the vagina between periods or after intercourse. The GP refers her to a gynaecologist who conducts another examination, possibly under anaesthetic, and takes specimens of tissue for investigation, to determine the exact nature of the disease. Blood samples and diagnostic X-rays to show how well the kidneys are working will have helped map out the extent of the problem.

Only at this point is the patient sent to see the radiotherapist. But this stage is important because it is then that some patients feel things must be worse than they really are. Referral for radiation treatment is thought to mean their disease is inoperable and therefore incurable. This is totally wrong. Surgery in the case of this woman would mean removal of all the pelvic organs. This is extremely traumatic, and although patients may be cured by it, the price they pay is thought by most doctors to be too great.

In patients like this woman, radiotherapy can provide a better chance of cure than is offered by surgery alone – with some immediate side-effects, but with few long-term complications. When the radiotherapist meets the patient, this is the first and most important point to discuss. The radiotherapist will also explain the nature of the disease, what radiotherapy will achieve, how the treatment will be conducted, and how long it will take.

In general, carcinoma of the cervix is treated by the delivery of radiation either from an X-ray machine, or from very small radioactive rods placed in the womb itself. Often these two treatments – using an external source of radiation and an internal one – are combined. Radiotherapy from an X-ray machine is illustrated in figure 5.2. The machine may move around the patient, attacking the tumour with beams of radiation from various angles.

To do this effectively, the precise position of the tumour must be known. So the first step in any radiotherapy treatment is establishing the exact size and site of the tumour, and the organs it is next to. With this information, the X-ray beams can be directed so that they 'hit' the tumour, while avoiding important tissues. A precise outline is made of the patient, and X-ray pictures taken of her in a variety of positions – something which is usually

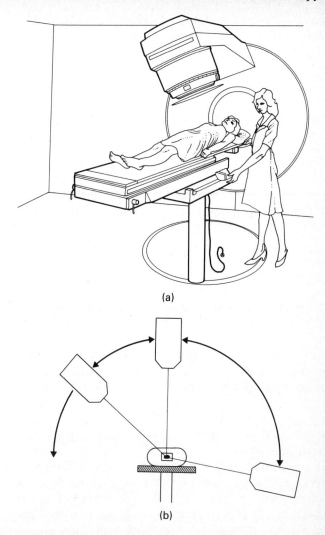

(a)

(b)

Figure 5.2 (a) A modern radiotherapy machine. By moving the couch and rotating the head of the machine, radiation is focused on the tumour. (b) Surrounding healthy tissue is spared un-necessary radiation. The machine does not come into contact with the patient.

done in a device, called a simulator, that exactly reproduces the conditions under which treatment will take
place. To help in the planning process, the radiotherapist
is able to study an X-ray image of the patient's internal
organs on a television screen. This preparation is the most
technical part of the whole radiotherapy procedure, and
though it may seem strange if not explained properly, it is
painless, and far less trouble for the patient than the
anaesthetic and biopsy she will already have gone through
to establish the diagnosis.

When the radiotherapist has all the information he
needs, the patient can be told more precisely how long the
treatment will take and how often she needs to come to
the hospital. Radiotherapy is usually given daily from
Monday to Friday for a period of five to seven weeks. So,
around 30 separate treatments can be expected, each
lasting a few minutes.

Indelible ink is used to mark the patient's skin, showing
the place where treatment is to be directed for the dura-
tion of the radiotherapy course. Patients are asked not to
remove these marks under any circumstances. The radiotherapist will also give individual instructions about any
alterations that may be needed in normal habits. There
may be certain parts of the body that should not be
washed. If part of the bowel is to be irradiated, foods
which are highly-spiced, bulky and laxative are best
avoided. Certain forms of alcohol, usually spirits, are also
advised against.

The radiotherapist will explain the side-effects that the
patient may notice, and suggest how they can be reduced.
Treatment of the pelvis exposes the bowel to radiation.
So, after ten to 14 days, there may be slight diarrhoea and
some discomfort passing urine. Such symptoms are mostly
minor, but unnecessary anxiety can be avoided if they are
understood before treatment begins. If radiotherapy lasts
for more than two weeks, or if a large volume of the body
is exposed, general tiredness may be another side-effect

of treatment. Though some patients are affected much more than others, all patients are best advised to rest as much as possible. But the precise advice given will depend on the patient and the type of therapy being used.

It is clear that most symptoms are made worse by anxiety, and that most anxiety arises from uncertainty. A patient who feels unclear about any aspect of treatment should ask the doctor. There is usually a good explanation for anything that may happen.

The patient can expect to see the radiotherapist at least once a week. He will check that the radiation 'prescription' is being correctly applied, and that no unexpected side-effects are occurring. Blood samples are taken to ensure problems, such as anaemia, do not develop. The radiotherapist is in overall charge. Treatment is given according to the radiotherapist's plan by radiographers, who are technicians trained specifically in the use of radiation therapy. Patients can be confident that everyone's efforts are directed towards making certain all is well.

Hyperthermia

X-rays have been used in the treatment of cancer for over 80 years. For almost as long, doctors have wondered whether cancer could also be treated by heat therapy, or hyperthermia. Sufficiently high temperatures will kill all cells, but there are good reasons to think that cancer cells are more sensitive to heat than their normal counterparts. The most important is that the blood vessels within tumours do not respond in the same way as the blood vessels in healthy tissue. The flow of blood is less, so the tumour is not so effectively cooled down, and greater damage can be expected.

Originally, at the turn of the century, the idea was that the temperature of the whole body should be raised by infecting the patient with an organism that produced fever, or by immersing him in a bath of hot liquid. These

techniques were unsatisfactory because the difference between the temperature of the tumour and that of the
surrounding healthy tissue was small. The idea of hyper-
themia was also overtaken by dramatic advances in the
1920s and 1930s in our ability to use X-rays for effective
treament. But interest in hyperthermia has recently re-
emerged.

Hyperthermia also involves a form of radiation, though
the rays that cause heating are more like the heat waves
produced in a microwave oven than the X-rays used in
radiotherapy. Tumours exposed to high temperatures
appear to shrink. They are not 'burned up' in the usual
sense of the term, since the temperature inside the
tumour reach only 42–45 degrees centigrade, a mere five
to eight degrees above normal body temperature. But the
fact that tumours withstand heat less well than normal
tissues means that their cells are selectively killed. Hyperthermia is being increasingly used in the United States,
and Britain has recently had its first machines installed. It
is too early to say how effective the new form of treatment
will be.

From the scientific standpoint, the encouraging aspect
of hyperthermia is that it works in a way entirely different
from X-rays. Cells which are deprived of oxygen, and so
resistant to radiotherapy, are sensitive to heat. This
means that hyperthermia and X-rays can be used
together, perhaps having an effect very much greater than
that produced by either method alone. The combination
of hyperthermia with drug therapy offers a similar hope.

6   Drug Treatment

We have seen how cancer confined to a particular area can be effectively treated by surgery and modern radiotherapy. Sadly, since cancer has often spread beyond its original site by the time it is discovered, these treatments may not be enough to produce a cure. This spread may be through direct invasion of healthy tissue by the tumour, or by small clumps of tumour cells breaking off and being carried away to other sites. Whether these migrating cells set up secondary cancers, or metastases, depends on factors that are discussed in chapter 1.

Once cancer has spread widely, so that it affects many systems within the body, the form of treatment used must also be systemic. In practice, this generally means treatment by drugs. These may be either hormones that mimic the body's natural chemical messengers which control the growth of certain kinds of cell, or drugs – called cytotoxics – that kill cancer cells. There are certain tumours (cancer of the breast being the most obvious example) that can be controlled, at least partly, by hormonal agents. The role of hormones is considered in a separate section at the end of this chapter. But for the majority of cancers, and often even for hormone-dependent tumours, the most successful form of systemic treatment is with cytotoxic drugs. Cytotoxics are frequently effective. The disadvantage is that they also have serious side-effects.

For many years, physicians and scientists have tried to

identify drugs that destroy cancer cells. Many have now been found. But the fundamental problem is one of selectivity. To be effective, an anti-cancer drug must kill tumour cells but leave their normal counterparts undamaged. The special problem posed by cancer can be understood if we consider a form of drug therapy – the use of antibiotics – that has been very successful in curing a different kind of disease.

In 1928, working in a small and rather dirty laboratory at St Mary's Hospital in Paddington, Alexander Fleming was studying bacteria growing on plates of broth. One of the plates became accidentally contaminated with a fungus, and Fleming noticed that the bacteria did not grow around the areas of contamination. The cause was a substance secreted by the bacteria. It was identified, and called penicillin. Although reported in a medical journal, Fleming's observation lay dormant for over ten years until Howard Florey, an Oxford scientist, realised the potential of the fungus as a way of treating patients who were infected with bacteria.

Penicillin is a remarkably non-toxic drug. It causes no side-effects until very high doses are reached; and long before this, bacteria causing the infection are killed. Research since then has revealed the way penicillin works. Unlike our own cells, bacteria are surrounded by a cell wall made of sugar proteins. Production of this cell wall requires certain biochemical processes, and penicillin prevents one of these from occurring. Since animal cell walls do not have a sugar protein coat, the drug has no adverse effects on our own cells and so does not cause problems when given to patients.

The discovery of penicillin and related drugs led to the eradication of infectious diseases as a major cause of death in the western world. Bacteria periodically develop ways of countering the effects of these drugs, but pharmacologists have so far always succeeded in staying one step ahead by devising new compounds to overcome drug resistance.

We are now looking for a drug that will be as significant a breakthrough for cancer treatment as the discovery of penicillin was for the treatment of infectious disease. The difficulty, though, is much greater. Bacteria are invading, 'foreign' organisms: their cells are quite different from our own. The problem with cancer is that tumour cells are derived from their normal counterparts. We have not yet discovered any biochemical process possessed by a cancer cell that is not also possessed by a normal cell at some stage of its development.

Cancer cells are measurably different in many ways. For example, the turnover of DNA within the nucleus of the cell is greater. This means the processes that produce the DNA building blocks, and the rate at which the cell divides, are faster. So too are the processes that form the strands to 'pull' the chromosomes apart. But these are differences in the rate at which various processes take place. They are not differences in the type of process.

How do anti-cancer drugs work?

At the moment, the one way we can tackle cancer cells is to make use of the fact that they reproduce rapidly. Though there is no single drug which is effective against all types of cancer, there are chemicals making use of this difference that kill particular types of tumour cells.

The individual drugs that are most frequently used in the treatment of cancer, and their different effects, are described towards the end of the chapter. Ultimately, they all work through stopping cell division. Since healthy cells also divide, these drugs have side-effects, many of which are unavoidable. The normal cells that are worst affected are those that divide rapidly. Such cells are found in the bone marrow, the hair follicles, skin, and the lining of the intestines.

The discovery of anti-cancer drugs

It is ironic that the first drug successfully used against human cancer was a by-product of research into chemical warfare. During the First World War, scientists developed a variety of compounds which caused severe irritation to the skin and eyes. We now know these chemicals acted by becoming attached to DNA in certain cells in the skin and cornea. They also severely damaged the lungs.

As part of the development programme, the compounds were given to volunteers in non-lethal doses. Blood samples were taken, and it was quickly noticed that a major effect was a very rapid fall in the number of white blood cells. One of the chemicals investigated was mustard gas, containing a substance called nitrogen mustard, which had an especially severe effect on the white cell count.

Towards the end of the Second World War, the American pharmacologist Louis Goodman was trying to develop drugs to treat lymphoma, a form of cancer in which the white cells reproduce out of control. He realised that if nitrogen mustard could reduce the number of normal white cells, it might reduce the number of cancerous white cells also. A patient with lymphoma was treated with a single injection of mustine. Within a few days, the enlarged lymph nodes under the armpits and in the groin, which are the most important signs of the disease, had disappeared. Unfortunately, the nodes became enlarged again four weeks later. Another injection of mustine was given. Again the nodes disappeared, but again returned, and the patient eventually died of the disease. But his good initial response to the drug was the first clear demonstration that a chemical compound could have profound anti-cancer effects in a patient.

The discovery gave new impetus to the search for a chemical cure. In Boston, in the early 1950s, a drug which inhibited the creation of the building blocks of DNA was synthesised. The compound, methotrexate, was found useful in treating children with leukaemia. Although few children were cured with methotrexate alone, many had their lives significantly prolonged. This second demonstration that tumour cells could be destroyed within the human body again intensified research efforts.

The drug industry, cancer institutes and universities all over the world began testing chemical compounds for their effectiveness against tumour cells grown in the laboratory. Drugs which killed cells in this initial screening were then used in mice and rats in whom tumours had been artificially induced. Many of the compounds were similar to the nitrogen mustards and methotrexate, but totally new substances were also discovered.

Few of these drugs could be shown to cure patients. Although they significantly reduced the amount of tumour present, they did not eradicate tumour cells completely. Then, in 1965, the National Cancer Institute in Washington set up a new trial of drug therapy in patients who had another form of lymphatic cancer, called Hodgkin's disease. It was decided to treat patients simultaneously with four drugs known to be of some help individually, in the hope that their combined effects would produce a cure.

The four drugs – nitrogen mustard, vincristine, procarbazine and prednisone – were given over a fortnight. Two were given in tablet form every day, and the others by injection on the first and eighth day. Called MOPP after the initial letters of the four drugs (the trade name for vincristine is 'Oncovin'), the combination resulted in the complete and permanent disappearance of cancer from many patients. Many people who received MOPP in 1965 for widespread Hodgkin's disease are still alive.

This breakthrough was dramatic. It led to interest in new approaches, combining existing agents for a whole range of different cancer types. Over the next decade, four different types of cancer – lymphoma, testicular teratoma, choriocarcinoma and childhood leukaemia – became curable in many patients. The success was real, but very incomplete. Some people with these diseases still died. There were difficulties in the use of the drugs because of their side-effects. And there also emerged the problem of drug resistance. But the greatest disappointment was the relative insensitivity of some of the most common types of cancer (such as those of the lung, breast and colon) to the drugs that were so useful in tackling other, relatively rare tumours. Twenty years later, we are still looking for a drug treatment of these common cancers that will be as successful as the MOPP combination.

Side-effects

Anti-cancer drugs have profound side-effects because of the damage they do to normal cells. The first problem is sickness. This ranges from mild nausea to severe vomiting, which may occur within a few minutes of the injection of an anti-cancer drug. Patients may even start to vomit when they arrive in the hospital, long before they are given the drug. Occasionally, the association of a particular context with the effects of the drug is so strong that patients are sick when they see a white-coated doctor on television. These side-effects which occur in the absence of the drug are called 'psychogenic'.

To some extent, the problem can be controlled by an injection of other, anti-nausea, drugs given before the cytotoxic agent is injected. Tablets can also be taken to combat nausea, which may last several hours after treatment, though pills are of course little use if there is actual vomiting. In this case, a suppository, which allows the drug to be absorbed through the rectum, can be particularly helpful.

Some anti-cancer drugs cause worse nausea than others. Cisplatinum, used very successfully to treat cancer of the testis, causes particular problems. Patients given this drug are usually admitted to hospital and take sedatives to prevent the onset of sickness, which is almost inevitable.

Around ten years ago, in California, it was noticed that the smoking of marijuana seemed to alleviate the nausea produced by anti-cancer drugs. Studies were set up to isolate the active ingredient in the cannabis plant, and a drug derived from it is now used when vomiting is severe.

Nausea is extremely unpleasant for the patient. But from the medical point of view the effect of anti-cancer drugs on the bone marrow is a more dangerous side-effect. It is this that limits the dose that can be given, and in some cases is probably the barrier that prevents cure. Bone marrow manufactures the red blood cells that carry oxygen round the body, and the white cells that fight infection by bacteria and viruses. It is also the source of a third type of blood cell – the platelets that clump together at the site of injury to halt bleeding.

Cytotoxic drugs can adversely affect the production of all three of these cells. If the number of red blood cells falls, the result is anaemia, and the patient feels tired and listless. Breathlessness may also develop when there are too few cells to carry oxygen to the tissues. But production of red blood cells is relatively resistant to the effects of chemotherapy. Problems with the white cells and platelets are more likely. If the white cell count drops, susceptibility to infection is increased. Often, the organisms that cause problems are the bacteria normally present on our skin and in our mouths and throats, which intact body defences cope with quite adequately. If platelets fall, the clotting mechanism is impaired, and the patient may bleed from the nose, lungs and intestines.

All of these problems can be dealt with. The first step is to keep a careful check on the production of cells by the bone marrow. Anyone receiving chemotherapy has freqent blood samples taken, so that the levels of blood components can be measured. This is what is meant by a 'blood count'. If the count of any of these cells starts to fall, the chemotherapy given can be adjusted to reduce the adverse effect on the marrow. If the problem continues, the blood constituents affected can be directly restored by transfusion. When red cells are missing, the transfusion is of 'whole' blood. For white cell and platelet deficiencies, only these components are replaced. (The cells are extracted from large quantities of donated blood.) Infections that develop because of a fall in white cells are also treated with antibiotics.

The effect of cytotoxic drugs on the number of white blood cells is one reason patients given chemotherapy have an increased risk of infection. But cytotoxic drugs also affect other parts of the immune system, so further impairing our ability to deal with invading bacteria, viruses and fungi. The most severe form of infection is septicaemia, when bacteria start to reproduce within the blood. (The fluid component of blood, called serum, contains all the nutrients bacteria need to grow.) The condition starts with flu-like symptoms, and a rise in temperature. But toxic products released by the bacteria then cause the circulation to fail: blood pressure drops, and death results unless there is prompt treatment with antibiotics and fluids to support the circulation.

The risk of septicaemia can be reduced by removing sources of potential infection. But the most important factor in reducing life-threatening complications is our greater experience in the use of cytotoxic drugs, which means that treatment can be adjusted to limit damage to the immune system. Except with the most intensive chemotherapy regimes, septicaemia is now fortunately rare.

Temporary baldness is a far less serious, but still disturbing, side-effect of chemotherapy. The degree of hair loss varies from one patient to another, and with the kind of cytotoxic drugs used. Adriamycin, for example, produces severe baldness, whereas vincristine on its own rarely has this effect. The problem – which can be anything from a patchy thinning of the hair to complete alopecia – affects both men and women, and tends to appear around four weeks into a course of chemotherapy.

Baldness occurs because the cells within the hair follicle

are of a kind that divides rapidly, and so are affected by anti-cancer drugs. There have recently been attempts to control the extent of hair loss by reducing blood supply to the scalp at the time cytotoxic drugs are given, and in the period shortly afterwards, when the concentration of drug in the blood is highest. A tight band placed around the scalp, and the application of bags containing refrigerated fluid, are both ways of restricting blood supply. But they are inconvenient, and neither has proved very effective in preventing hair loss.

At the moment it is probably easier simply to accept that there will be temporary loss of hair, with the reassurance that it starts to regrow soon after the course of chemotherapy is stopped. The time taken to restore a full head of hair varies. After intensive drug treatment for teratoma, for example, a fuzz appears on the scalp within four weeks. By six months, hair has fully regrown. In the interim, cosmetic problems can be overcome by using a wig. Modern wigs that fit well and look realistic can be obtained either from the hospital or from shops. In some patients, eyebrows and pubic hair fall out during a course of chemotherapy. These areas of hair also regrow.

A further problem is that chemotherapy affects fertility. One cause is the natural reduction in sex drive which accompanies illness and unpleasant treatment. This is temporary: sex drive returns once treatment has ended. But there is also a direct effect of cytotoxic drugs on the ovaries and testes. Developing sperm can be damaged even by mild chemotherapy. Fewer sex cells are produced, and those that do form may be abnormal. This limits the chances of conception. The menstrual cycle may also be abolished, in which case ova are no longer released, and fertilisation is not possible.

Because of the damaging effects of chemotherapy on sex cells, physicians recommend that patients wait for at least two years from the time drug treatment ends before they try to have children. For women particularly, this makes good sense. If a cancer is going to return, and so require further treatment, this will usually happen within the first two years. Beyond that time, it is less likely further treatment will be needed, and the sperm and ova will once more be in a healthy condition. Chemotherapy is almost never given during pregnancy because of its damaging effects on the foetus.

Since cytotoxic drugs damage sex cells, chemotherapy might be expected to lead to a higher risk that babies will be born with abnormalities – even if the parents have waited for two years. In practice, this rarely occurs. Many children have now been born to parents who received chemotherapy, and there is no evidence that the risk of abnormality is greater.

Most people who have received chemotherapy return to normal fertility. But there is a chance that they will become sterile. The problem is more common among males, which (in a sense) is fortunate, since sperm can easily be stored. If particularly aggressive chemotherapy is being planned, and the man wishes to have children later, a sample of sperm is taken, mixed in a special medium containing protein and egg yolk, and frozen in liquid nitrogen at −176 degrees centigrade. At this temperature, sperm can be stored indefinitely. If it is needed, it is slowly thawed and used for artificial insemination. Sperm banks are now widely available.

Apart from the general side-effects on rapidly dividing but healthy cells, individual cytotoxic drugs may damage particular organs in the body. Adriamycin, for example, binds to heart muscle cells, and may eventually cause heart failure – though this is not usually a problem now that doctors are aware of the risk.

In the case of bleomycin, the organ at risk is the lung. Everyone given the drug is affected to some extent, but the problem is severe in only around 5 per cent of patients. The base of the lung starts to thicken, and the air-filled sacs fill with fluid containing white blood cells. Later, there is development of fibrous tissue, which shows on X-rays as scarring of the lungs. At this stage patients may find that breathlessness interferes with their ability to move around. Fortunately these lung changes disappear with time. Within a year of ending treatment, even the most sensitive measures of lung function have returned to normal. With methotrexate, it is the liver that may be affected. If damage occurs, a great range of the body's biochemical processes are disrupted. But the chances of this happening are significant only if high doses of the drug have to be used.

The question of infertility arises only because chemotherapy has made such a contribution to the treatment of certain forms of cancer. Previously, patients would not have been expected to survive long enough for their future fertility to be considered a problem. The same is true of the possibility that patients given particular cytotoxic drugs may develop a second malignancy.

It is now clear that patients treated for lymphoma in the late 1960s, using a particular early combination of radiotherapy and chemotherapy, have a chance of developing leukaemia which is greater than would be expected. It takes many years for cancer to develop; so this is a problem which has only recently come to light. And even with this increase in risk, the likelihood that an ex-patient will develop leukaemia is still very small, and is obviously outweighed by the benefits of treatment.

As chemotherapy becomes more successful still, it may be that the occurrence of a second cancer – many years later – will become a problem. This is one reason much research effort is directed at finding the smallest possible dose of cytotoxic drugs that is effective. If the quantity of drugs given can be reduced, there will also be fewer immediate side-effects, and less likelihood of difficulties with fertility.

The complications discussed so far are physical. But there may also be psychological consequences. One of them is the development of dependence on the hospital and its staff. Given the unpleasant nature of the treatment, it is surprising – but true – that some patients find it difficult to accept that no further chemotherapy is needed, even after they are cured. This feeling of dependence must have its roots in the intensity of the experience, and the care that accompanies it.

But it is much more usual for people to find chemotherapy distressing. Some feel they cannot carry on and complete a planned course of treatment. Realising that their problems are faced by everyone who undergoes this form of therapy often helps. So too does having the cause of the problems explained. Frank discussion between the patient and doctor is often sufficient to allay the worst fears. Patients who can withstand a full course of treatment have a greater chance of recovery; and it is important that no-one gives up chemotherapy because they feel that they alone are experiencing difficulties.

Can chemotherapy cure?

There are certain cancers for which chemotherapy is undoubtedly a cure. They include testicular cancer and Hodgkin's disease. The tumour disappears completely, and does not return. But it is equally true that currently available chemotherapy offers little prospect of cure in some other cancers. The disease can be held in check for a while, and perhaps reversed, but it then progresses despite the continued use of a variety of drugs.

One of the major problems is drug resistance. Certain types of lung cancer, for example, are initially very sensitive even to small doses of cytotoxic drugs; but after six months the disease recurs, and this time it is resistant to everything that can be thrown at it.

The development of drug resistance is evolution in miniature: the 'fittest' cells survive. Even within the same tumour, cancer cells differ slightly in their genetic make-up in ways that affect their ability to withstand the onslaught of cytotoxic drugs. The cells that are suspectible die, or at least stop dividing; those that are not, survive and outstrip their neighbours in growth. In this way, clones of drug resistant cells evolve. We will probably not be able to make significant progress in dealing with this problem until we have a better understanding of the genetic mechanisms involved in the development of drug resistance.

But even in the solid tumours that do not respond well to chemotherapy, the use of cytotoxic drugs has a part to play in limiting the spread of the disease and extending life. In breast cancer, for example, disease that has spread to the chest wall can often be eradicated by the skilful use of drugs. But if the doctor and patient accept that the aim of chemotherapy is palliation of the disease rather than cure, their attitude to the side-effects of treatment may be different. In patients with Hodgkin's disease and teratoma, for example, aggressive therapy is justified even in people whose cancer is widespread. The chances of cure are very good, and the unpleasantness of treatment is an acceptable price to pay. But in other cancers the position may be different.

One of the most difficult dilemmas facing a physician is knowing when to stop active treatment. In recent years, full discussion between patients and doctors has helped to make clear that as far as the well-being of the patient is concerned, there are limits to the pursuit of cure. If the chances are not good, and the side-effects are severe, consideration of the whole patient – rather than simply of the disease – may suggest that use of aggressive drug treatment is not appropriate.

Some common cytotoxic drugs

No specific drug, or way of giving it, is the one 'right' treatment for any particular form of cancer. The reasons for using a specific therapy in an individual case can only be fully explained in discussion between the doctor and patient involved.

Cytotoxic drugs are often given in combination. Several drugs may be given together, usually in short bursts. The reason is that the bone marrow, the organ least tolerant of chemotherapy, can recover in the interval between successive courses, while the tumour cannot. Certain cytotoxic drugs have been designed by pharmaceutical chemists to have a specific anti-cancer action. Others were identified by routine testing of a wide range of existing compounds, or discovered as naturally occurring plant products.

Adriamycin was found when screening the products of fungi. It is said its name derives from that the fact the fungus was first identified growing on a castle overlooking the Adriatic sea. Adriamycin is a large molecule that works by binding to the DNA within cells, so reducing cell division and the production of proteins.

It is usually given every three weeks in combination with other drugs. Adriamycin is very irritant and so is given intravenously into a vein in the arm, rather than by mouth. Even with intravenous use, great care has to be taken. If any drug escapes from the vein, perhaps because the blood vessel wall is fragile, an unpleasant ulcer can be produced. When diluted, adriamycin has a bright red colour, and is sometimes known by patients as the 'red devil'. The most common side-effect is baldness, which occurs in everyone given the drug. But a more important problem is that high doses may affect the heart.

Bleomycin, discovered 20 years ago, is also produced by a fungus. It was isolated in Japan, where it was found to be particularly effective against lymphoma. More recently it has come to be used in combination with other drugs in the treatment of testicular cancer. Bleomycin is not irritant and can be given by injection intravenously, under the skin, or into muscle. But it is not given as a tablet because its absorption from the stomach is uncertain. The main side-effect specific to this drug is the possibility of a severe lung inflammation leading to fibrosis. Bleomycin also causes darkening of the skin, especially around scars. Any scratch marks also become pigmented, though no-one knows the reason. All these side-effects start to disappear as soon as the drug course is ended.

Chlorambucil is an alkylating agent, that is it binds to the bases of the DNA molecule, cross-linking them and so inhibiting cell division. Chlorambucil is one of the easiest anti-cancer drugs to use since it can be given orally. Tablets are usually taken daily, either continuously or for two weeks followed by a two-week gap – to allow the bone marrow to recover, so making the tumour-damaging effect of the drug more selective.

Cyclophosphamide is also an alkylating agent, which was designed to be changed into its active form by the enzymes in tumours. It can be given by mouth or by injection. About 20 seconds after the drug is injected into a vein, the patient may experience a metallic taste, as the drug circulates rapidly and the taste buds are stimulated. Another side-effect is irritation of the lining of the bladder, caused by a breakdown by-product. In a few patients, this may lead to the appearance of blood in the urine. Cyclophosphamide is used mostly in lymphoma, breast and ovarian cancer.

Cisplatinum was discovered 20 years ago, completely by accident. A scientist investigating the effects of electrical fields on bacteria noticed that a current passing between platinum electrodes slowed the rate of bacterial growth. Later studies showed that if the fluid left at the end of the experiment was poured onto a fresh batch of bacteria, they were killed. This suggested it was not the electric current itself that was having the effect, but small amounts of platinum released from the electrode.

The drug which was developed from this discovery turned out to have anti-cancer properties, and it is now widely used in treating testicular and ovarian cancer. Cisplatinum is also being investigated as a possible treatment for a range of other tumours. Use of the drug is complicated by its effects on the kidneys. To counter this side-effect, a high intake of fluids is needed.

5-Fluorouracil, which can be given either by mouth or by injection, is useful in some patients with cancer of the breast, colon and rectum, and other malignancies of the gastro-intestinal tract. In normal doses, it is one of the least upsetting anti-cancer drugs.

Methotrexate, one of the oldest cytotoxic drugs, inhibits the action of a series of cell enzymes responsible for making the building blocks of DNA. In doing so, it slows the growth of cells that divide frequently, and so have a rapid turnover of DNA. The tendency to develop severe mouth ulcers, with the risk that they become infected, is a side-effect peculiar to this drug. It can be given in tablet form or intravenously.

Methotrexate is unusual in that a very powerful anti-dote, folinic acid, is available. There have been attempts to see if high doses of methotrexate, followed 24 hours later by the antidote, increase the number of tumour cells killed, whilst sparing the bone marrow.

Certain bone cancers, particularly in young people, seem especially responsive to this method of administering the drug.

Vincristine and Vinblastine are drugs with very similar properties that come from the periwinkle, a plant with small purple flowers, common in many English gardens. Whole fields of the plants are harvested and sent to pharmaceutical firms for the drug to be extracted. Both drugs, in combination with other agents, are effective against lymphomas and a variety of other tumours.

Vincristine is less toxic to the bone marrow than vinblastine, but affects the nerves that carry signals to and from the hands and feet, producing tingling and possibly numbness in the fingers and toes. Vincristine may also produce pain in the jaw which is sometimes serious enough to produce spasm of the main jaw muscles. Both drugs are given by intravenous injection since they are not absorbed from the intestine.

Use of these drugs is not exclusive to cancer. Their action in slowing excessive cell division can also be helpful in other conditions. Cyclophosphamide, for example, is used to suppress the action of lymphocytes after organ transplantation, so reducing the chances of rejection; and small doses of methotrexate are valuable in treating the skin disease psoriasis.

Hormones

Hormones are chemical messengers. They became necessary during evolution as animals increased in size. In a single-celled organism, such as the amoeba, simple diffusion of chemicals within the cell is sufficient to co-ordinate the activities of its various parts. But as animals grew larger, and groups of cells came to have specialised functions, some form of communication between the various organs became necessary. The nervous system evolved as a way of passing information quickly from one part of the body to another. Complementary to that, there arose another mechanism to deal with longer-term control, especially of the growth and development of organs. This was the system of endocrine, or hormone-producing glands.

The endocrine glands include the pituitary at the base of the brain, the thyroid in the neck, the adrenals above the kidneys, and the ovaries and testes. Many of the hormones produced by these organs regulate the growth of specific tissues. For example, the female sex hormone oestrogen, produced by the ovaries, stimulates growth of certain cells in the breast. The androgens, in men, stimulate the growth of tissue in the prostate. Hormones can also inhibit the growth of cells.

In 1896, George Beatson, a Scottish surgeon, removed the ovaries of two young patients with advanced breast cancer. In both women, the disease began to regress. Though the tumours later returned, this was the first demonstration that changing the levels of hormones circulating in the body could be effective against cancer. We now know the that removal of the ovaries leads to a fall in levels of oestrogen in the blood. The amount of oestrogen reaching the breast tumour is therefore less, and the rate of division of cancer cells is reduced. Since then hormonal therapy has been widely used for cancers arising in tissues susceptible to hormonal influence. They include tumours of the breast, prostate, uterus, and kidney.

There are three ways levels of a hormone, and its effects, can be influenced. The first is to destroy or make ineffective the endocrine gland that produces it. This can be done by surgery, radiation or drugs. Any of these three methods can be used to treat the ovaries, for example – though the treatment will of course not be used in women who are well past child-bearing age. With the menopause, production of oestrogen gradually falls over a period of a few years.

The second approach is to *give* a hormone. This may mean exceptionally large doses of a substance the body produces naturally: unusually high levels of a hormone can inhibit cell growth even though the naturally occurring levels stimulate it. Patients with breast cancer therefore sometimes receive extra oestrogen. Alternatively, the hormone given may be one that the body would not normally secrete, but which happens to have the desired effect on a tumour. This is the case when prostate cancers in men are treated with large doses of the female hormone oestrogen.

The third technique is to develop drugs that prevent hormones reaching their target. Hormones, and other chemicals with biological effects, can be thought of as keys. To have an effect, they must fit into locks, which are found in the form of receptors, on the surface (or within) a cell. If another substance fits the same lock, that is, occupies the receptor, the hormone may be prevented from exerting its usual effects. These blocking drugs are often called anti-hormones. The best example of an anti-hormone is tamoxifen, which blocks the action of oestrogen and so is widely used in the treatment of breast cancer.

The effect of tamoxifen is direct. But hormone levels can be manipulated in a more roundabout way. A good example of this is use of drugs that affect the pituitary gland, which is sometimes described as 'the conductor of the endocrine orchestra'. Many endocrine organs work under a complicated hierarchy of controls. They are often influenced by the pituitary gland which itself receives instructions from part of the brain known as the hypothalamus. Recently a variety of agents has been developed to block the signals that pass from the hypothalamus to the pituitary. These 'releasing-factor analogues' can have a profound effect on the levels of circulating hormones. Their use in breast and prostate cancer is being carefully investigated.

It should be emphasised that not all patients respond to hormone treatment. Even among cancers arising from the same tissue, the response to hormones is variable, and depends on how richly the tumour cells are supplied with hormone receptors. The number of receptors can be measured by taking a small sample of cancer tissue. This test is sometimes used to assess the chances that hormone therapy will produce good results.

But hormone treatment has relatively few side-effects. There is no depression of the bone marrow or loss of hair. Indeed, in some cases, hormones may act as a tonic. In all patients who have a tumour that arises in a hormone-dependent organ there is a good chance of response to hormone therapy. For these reasons, hormones are often used as a worthwhile first treatment in the full range of patients.

7   Different Types of Cancer

Although a malignant tumour that starts in one organ may spread to many others, it is the organ or tissue where the cancer begins that gives its name to the disease as a whole. So if a cancer of the breast spreads to form secondary tumours in the bones, it is still referred to as breast cancer. This way of describing tumours is useful because cancers that arise in a particular organ behave in a similar way. Doctors therefore know which symptoms to look out for, and which tests to perform. For example, tumours starting in a man's prostate gland tend to spread to bones, so that development of bone pain in a patient with prostate cancer may be an important symptom. It is less likely to be significant in a patient whose primary tumour is of the lymphatic system, since this cancer only rarely spreads to affect the bones. A doctor would therefore look for some other cause of the bone pain.

Figure 7.1 shows the organs of the body that are most frequently affected by cancer, in men and women. In this chapter, certain of the more common forms of cancer are described in greater detail. By understanding how these cancers usually develop (something which is termed their 'natural history') it should become clear why doctors ask certain questions, and why they examine certain organs particularly carefully. Doctors do not perform tests for the sake of doing them. Clinical investigations are expen-

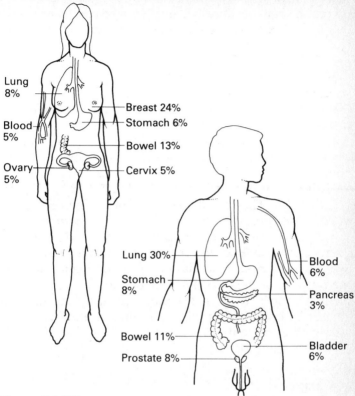

Figure 7.1 Where common tumours occur. Percentages show the proportion of all cancer accounted for by tumours at each site.

sive, and time-consuming. So, lying behind every investigation, is a question that needs an answer.

A point to bear in mind is that this chapter often describes what happens if the disease is left untreated. The aim of therapy is to slow the progress of the illness, and if possible to halt or even reverse the disease. So what happens to an individual patient will hopefully be different from what would have happened if the disease had not been tackled.

Nevertheless, to give a fair account, the failures of current therapy must be presented alongside its successes. Only by understanding why some treatments do not work will we be able to improve on them. Even with the remarkable success stories, some of which are described in this chapter, there is a cost to pay in side-effects. Some reading may therefore be painful and depressing. But that is the nature of the disease, and of our incomplete ability to deal with it.

It is not possible fully to describe each kind of cancer. There will be many exceptions to all the situations outlined in this book. But, even in the few paragraphs devoted to each form of cancer, the general principles can be explained. They should be sufficient to aid understanding of what is happening, and why. This type of explanation is not a substitute for detailed discussion with the doctor responsible for the care of an individual patient. In every case of cancer the nature of the particular disease, the purpose of the tests performed, and the aim of treatment will need to be considered afresh by the medical adviser in consultation with the patient, and his or her family. We can only present the central facts on which such discussion can be based.

Curability

In everyday speech, the terms 'curable' and 'incurable' are often applied to cancer. These terms have their use, but can be misleading. Cancer is a complicated disease, and simple labels do not always fit.

With few exceptions, cancer is a chronic illness, and the course of the disease may last several years, even without treatment. There are forms of cancer which are incurable in the strict sense of the term, but which develop so slowly that the patient has many years of normal life in prospect. In certain types of thyroid cancer, usually those developing in young women, it is not uncommon for patients to live for 30 years after metastatic disease has been diagnosed. Chronic lymphatic leukaemia is another cancer which can be so mild in its effects that treatment is given only when specific symptoms, such as painfully swollen lymph glands, occur. In both these examples, the patient is not cured of the disease, and is in fact incurable in the sense that we cannot say all malignant cells have been banished from the body. But this can still be compatible with long survival and a good quality of life.

The concept of cure is also of only limited use in the case of a disease like breast cancer in which secondary deposits of tumour can lie dormant and unsuspected for years. Even when the tumour becomes active again, it can often be controlled by therapy for a further long period.

For a cancer to be incurable does not necessarily mean that the patient will quickly die of the disease, nor even that he or she will die of it at all. Cancer becomes much more common with age. A person aged 70 with chronic cancer may be as likely to die of some unrelated problem, such as a heart attack, as of their malignant disease.

This fact is reflected in a problem with official statistics relating to cause of death. Although a cause must be written on all death certificates, so that the impact of different diseases can be assessed, figures that are based on this information can be misleading. We are not told how long the disease that caused death had been present, nor how well it had been controlled by treatment. Some epidemiologists believe that doctors are too ready to list cancer as the cause of death in all patients who are known at some stage to have experienced the disease. Cancer may be cited when the real cause of death was some other problem. If true, this would lead to an unnecessarily pessimistic assessment of the chances of surviving cancer.

A further complication is that age affects not only the likelihood that cancer will develop, but also the character of the disease.

Some forms of tumour, such as breast cancer, are less aggressive in older patients than in younger ones; but others, such as cancer of the oesophagus, become more severe in their effect. It should also be remembered that an older person, who has a variety of medical problems quite separate from cancer, may not be able to withstand treatment. So cancer may be the final illness in someone of advanced age, and will be recorded as the cause of death, even though in someone better able to tolerate treatment the disease might have been 'curable'.

These and other factors make it difficult to interpret cancer statistics. That difficulty, together with what seems to be a natural tendency to remember cases that fared badly rather than those that did well, helps explain some of the (perhaps unnecessary) fear that cancer arouses.

Skin cancer

The commonest cancers are those of the skin. But treatment is so remarkably successful that most official statistics do not even record the number of cases that occur. The main exception to this is melanoma, a cancer arising in the pigment cells deep within the skin. Attention is paid to this form of cancer because it is the most difficult to treat successfully.

Cancers which start in the skin seem to have the same cause – ultraviolet light. For this reason, skin tumours are more common in people exposed to sunlight and on parts of the body, such as the face, that are not protected by clothes. In Britain, farmers and other outdoor workers are the most frequently affected. Fair-skinned people living in tropical climates also appear to be susceptible.

Tumours called basal cell carcinomas, or 'rodent ulcers' are the most common form of skin cancer. The association with rodents arises because the cancer, if left untreated, 'eats' away at the surrounding tissue. If neglected, basal cell carcinomas can become larger. But the disease is unique amongst malignant tumours in not spreading to other parts of the body. If tackled early enough, all rodent ulcers can be eradicated by radiation. Those that have been neglected are more difficult. But even they can often be cured by surgery – though extensive treatment, and the use of skin grafts, is sometimes necessary.

The second most common skin cancers are tumours of the deeper, squamous cell layer of the skin. They usually occur on the face or hands, and take the form of hard, irregul. ulcers. If ignored, squamous cell carcinomas can spread to nearby lymph nodes. As with most tumours, smaller growths can be cured more easily than larger ones. Depending on where on the body they occur, the most appropriate treatment may be either radiotherapy or surgery. In the case of larger tumours it is usual to deal with the surrounding lymph nodes at the same time, either by removing them surgically or by including them in the area to be irradiated.

Melanoma is the most serious form of skin tumour. This is a cancer of the pigment-containing cells that give skin its colour. The tumours formed may be very dark, even black. They are sometimes difficult to distinguish from ordinary moles, and for this reason doctors advise the removal of any mole which changes size or shape, or which bleeds. Melanoma is treated principally by surgery. Smaller growths can be dealt with very adequately. But melanomas tend to metastasise more widely than any other skin tumour. A common site for spread is the liver. If this occurs, chemotherapy (that is treatment with cytotoxic drugs that kill cancer cells) is required. In addition to standard chemotherapy, other drugs that stimulate the immune system have been used with some success against the disease.

Lung cancer

Cancer of the lung is the most frequently fatal cancer. It is a sad irony, since this is the form of cancer that we could do most to prevent. For over 20 years we have known that cigarette smoking is by far the most important cause; yet millions of people continue to smoke.

There is recent evidence that the death rate from lung cancer is beginning to fall among middle-aged men, and that its increase among women has stopped. This is due partly to the smaller number of people who smoke, and partly to the fact that almost all smokers have switched from high-tar unfiltered cigarettes to lower-tar brands with filter tips. But any reduction in risk in smoking filter cigarettes is small. The only way really to reduce the chance of getting lung cancer is not to smoke at all. Quitting smoking is difficult, and many people started on the addictive habit at a time when its dangers were not known. But the risk of lung cancer starts to diminish as soon as a person stops, and after ten to 15 years is back at the level of a non-smoker. Apart from lung cancer, cigarette smoking also causes cancer of the larynx, trachea and bladder and contributes to deaths from heart disease.

There are two reasons why lung cancer is such a serious disease. First, by the time the original primary tumour in the lung has grown large enough to cause symptoms, secondary spread to distant organs will almost certainly already have occurred. It is these secondaries that are most dangerous to the patient. Treating the primary lesion alone, by local measures such as surgery and radiotherapy, is therefore unlikely to be successful. And most forms of lung cancer (the exception is considered later) are not sensitive to the systemic drug treatments that are available. One reason patients with lung cancer delay consulting the doctor is that early symptoms such as cough, shortness of breath and chest pain are experienced by smokers as everyday events.

The second reason lung cancer is difficult to treat successfully is that most cases occur in elderly patients after a lifetime's cigarette smoking. Even if the cancer remained localised and could be removed by taking out one of the lungs, smoking's other adverse effects – such as chronic bronchitis and emphysema – mean that the remaining lung would probably not be healthy enough to support the patient. Smokers often also have heart disease, and their general condition is too poor for them to withstand the major surgery that might rid them of their disease.

Before embarking on surgery, the surgeon will need to be sure that the tumour can be cut out without damaging vital structures in the body, and that the remaining lung will work adequately on its own. This means that the patient with lung cancer will have his blood investigated, X-rays taken, and tests of lung function made in the build-up towards an operation.

If it is found that the tumour is small enough, but the general condition of the patient is too poor to allow surgery, very high doses of radiation can be given to a small area of tissue. This procedure, called radical radiotherapy, can produce results which are as good as surgery. Unfortunately, many tumours are too large for high-dose irradiation. In these circumstances, symptoms such as cough and pain can be reduced, but the tumour is not destroyed.

The most encouraging response to chemotherapy is seen in patients with a type of lung tumour known as small cell carcinoma. Though the tumour divides rapidly and may spread quickly through the chest and to other organs, it is the form of lung cancer most sensitive to drug treatment. There are a variety of drug combinations now available that shrink the tumour and greatly lengthen survival. Unfortunately, only 20 per cent of lung cancers are small cell carcinomas. But if we can learn more about this tumour, we may understand better what is happening in other forms of lung cancer and so devise more effective drug treatments for them also.

Breast cancer

One in 17 British women will develop a breast tumour at some time in their lives. Treatment is successful in early stages of the disease when the tumour is small, but is less effective as the cancer becomes advanced.

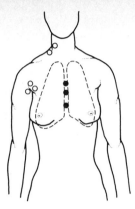

○ Superficial lymph nodes

● Deep lymph nodes

Figure 7.2 The position of lymph nodes within the chest, under the arm and at the base of the neck, that may be involved in breast cancer. Open circles show nodes near the surface of the skin; filled circles represent deep nodes.

The distinction between 'early' and 'advanced' refers to a stage in the biological development of the disease, rather than simply the length of time symptoms have been present, or the size of the tumour. 'Early' disease is confined to the breast, or extends only to the lymph nodes nearby. (Figure 7.2 shows the position of the lymph nodes that may be affected.) This stage of disease can be cured by surgery, radiotherapy or a combination of both. In 'advanced' disease, cancer has already spread to other organs. Although there is a relationship between the size of the tumour and the likelihood that the disease has spread, cancer may still be confined to the breast even when the primary tumour is large.

Contrary to popular belief, breast cancer is often a slow-growing tumour: many specialists think that malignant cells have been present for between five and ten years before a lump can first be felt. It makes sense to try to detect and treat the disease at the earliest possible point, ideally well before the tumour is large enough to become obvious to the woman herself – hence the importance of screening clinics. The need for early detection also makes routine self-examination an important aspect of cancer control. The screening clinics use a combination of skilled examination by hand, and very 'soft', low-dose X-rays to reveal suspicious lumps in women who show no signs of disease. The use of ultrasound (described in chapter 3) is also becoming important.

Because of the slow growth of breast tumours, many lengthy studies have been needed to show that screening clinics are leading to higher rates of cure. From what we know about the development of the disease, early detection should be an advantage, and the first firm evidence is now beginning to emerge.

When a woman goes to her doctor with a lump that can already be felt, the first stage is to establish whether the growth is benign or malignant. This is done by taking a small sample of tissue from the lump for examination under a microscope. If the growth proves to be cancerous, the doctor will need to assess the extent of tumour spread (if any has occurred) by a combination of physical examination and other investigations. (Further details of the biopsy procedure can be found in the chapter on diagnosis.)

Metastases will be discovered in only a few cases. But up to half the women who show no signs at this stage that the disease has spread will go on to develop secondary tumours. This means that metastases are present, even though they cannot be detected by the tests we use today. The best way to diagnose and treat these 'micro-metastases' is now being researched.

But the initial problem is the primary tumour. It has long been known that removal of the lump alone is not enough: in most cases, cancer simply develops again in the same place. Because of this, the surgeon William

Halsted developed a technique called 'radical mastectomy', at the end of the last century. This involves removal of the whole breast, plus the muscle and lymph nodes that lie under it. Although disfiguring, the operation is successful in preventing local recurrence of the disease.

It took many years of careful research to show that equally good results could be achieved by a less extensive operation, providing radiotherapy was used as well. This operation, termed simple mastectomy, preserves the underlying muscle of the chest wall. More recent studies have tended to show that increasing the dose of radiation means that the extent of surgery can be less again. Doctors now believe that removal of the lump and a wide margin of surrounding tissue, plus high-energy radiotherapy, is sufficient in many patients to prevent the cancer returning at its original site.

However, effective treatment of the primary tumour still leaves 50 per cent of women with hidden micro-metastases. It was as an attempt to eliminate them that the concept of adjuvant therapy was born. The idea is that use of anti-cancer drugs or hormones following radiotherapy and surgery might prevent women developing the disease that they are harbouring. The idea is sensible, but putting it into practice has caused controversy among cancer specialists.

Adjuvant chemotherapy using cytotoxic drugs can be useful. But the most effective drug regimes are the most complicated to administer, and have the highest incidence of side-effects. And though the onset of further disease can be delayed in many women, drugs appear to eradicate it in only a few. At present, we cannot identify who those few women will be; and many doctors feel they cannot justify subjecting large numbers of women to an unpleasant form of therapy when only a small proportion of them will benefit. Compared with their colleagues in Europe, American cancer specialists are more inclined to treat women with breast cancer by adjuvant chemotherapy, usually for a year. This is one example of how cancer therapy varies from one country to another, and demonstrates how doctors who have the same aim – complete cure of the patient, with the smallest amount of discomfort possible – can have honest differences of opinion about how best to achieve it.

The difficulty in using drugs as an adjuvant treatment of breast cancer arises because the only substances we have at present are so toxic. (Their effects are described in the chapter on chemotherapy.) If the drugs were more generally effective, and had fewer side-effects, more doctors would be prepared to offer treatment, and more patients to undergo it. There is hope that hormones may help provide an answer.

All breast tissue, whether normal or malignant, is sensitive to hormones – as is shown by the change in breast shape and size in the course of the menstrual cycle. To grow properly, breast tissue appears to need the female hormone, oestrogen. This suggests that hormones can play a part in treating breast cancer, and that the first priority is to reduce the presence or effectiveness of normal supplies of oestrogen. In menstruating women this can be most effectively accomplished by removing or irradiating the ovaries. The adrenal glands are the next most important source of oestrogens, and they are sometimes also treated by a drug which stops them functioning. These forms of hormone therapy can be very successful in patients with metastatic breast cancer, and are more fully described in the last section of the chapter on drug treatments.

The influence of oestrogen can also be reduced by an anti-hormone drug that blocks its effects. This drug is well established in the treatment of advanced disease. There is increasing evidence that it may also be useful as adjuvant therapy, that is for women who are apparently free of disease, but who we know run the risk that breast cancer will later return.

Whether or not adjuvant treatment is given, many women eventually develop secondary disease. What causes this to appear, sometimes many years after the primary cancer has been successfully treated, is not known. The metastases must have been present throughout the disease-free period, but somehow held in check by the patient's own defences. We are not at all clear what occurs to disturb the balance; but many oncologists believe factors such as severe psychological shock can play a part.

If disease recurs, several types of treatment can be useful, apart from the hormone therapy which has already been described. Radiotherapy can destroy small amounts of metastatic tumour which may be causing symptoms. And combination chemotherapy also has a place. But again the problem is that the most effective combinations are those with the most severe side-effects, and the time to use them must be very carefully evaluated in patients who may already be quite poorly.

Bowel cancer

Cancers occurring in the digestive passages, which stretch from the mouth to the rectum, are common. Certain parts of this continuous tube seem especially prone to tumours. These areas include the stomach and the lower part of the large bowel, or colon. But other sections of the digestive tract, such as the small bowel, which lies between the stomach and colon, are very rarely affected. (The large and small bowel, together, form the intestine.)

Tumours of the large bowel account for a large proportion of the cancers experienced by people in western countries, where they are responsible for around one in ten cancer deaths. But there is striking variation in the incidence of colon cancer in the world as a whole, and this should provide evidence about the causes of the disease. Colon tumours are rare in countries where the food eaten is largely unprocessed, and so has a high content of fibre – the undigestible remains of plant cell walls. Among rural Africans, for example, consumption of fibre is high, and large bowel cancer is infrequent.

The idea that lack of fibre in the typical western diet is responsible for our high rate of colon cancer was originally suggested by the British surgeon Denis Burkitt, who worked for many years in Africa and who has written widely about fibre and health. But the cause of colon cancer cannot simply be lack of fibre. The Eskimos, for example, eat hardly any fibre at all, and yet they too have little colon cancer. Nevertheless, there is probably something about our diet which is responsible, perhaps in association with exposure to carcinogenic chemicals in the environment. Recent evidence suggests particular ways of storing meat may contribute to the risk: though flavour is enhanced, levels of carcinogenic chemicals increase.

There is also a genetic susceptibility to the disease, at least in some patients. This is seen most clearly in people who have a condition called familial polyposis coli. The disease is inherited, and inevitably leads at some stage to colon cancer. But in patients whose colon starts off being normal, it is the environment that is involved in most cases of the disease. The best evidence for this is the experience of people who have migrated from one country to another, taking their genetic make-up with them, but altering their environment. Japanese who moved to the United States provide a striking example. In Japan, the colon cancer rate is about one-fifth that in the US. Yet Japanese immigrants in America quickly developed a very similar incidence of disease to that found in native Americans. If the cause of the change could only be identified, it could probably be avoided.

In Britain, the typical patient with colon cancer is aged over 55, and has a lifetime history of eating a standard western diet. There is little difference in incidence between men and women.

The tumour usually draws attention to itself by causing discomfort or pain in the lower abdomen. There may also be some alteration of bowel habit, particularly a tendency towards constipation. Discharge of mucus, and bleeding, are important warning signs.

Bowel cancer usually starts as an ulcer in the tissue forming the innermost layer of the intestine, and grows through the full thickness of the bowel wall. There may then be spread to the lymph nodes near the bowel, and to other, healthy organs in the pelvis. Spread to distant organs, such as the liver, occurs only at a late stage in the disease. For this reason, the main treatment for bowel cancer is surgical. An attempt is made to remove the tumour and adjacent portions of bowel, plus the nearby lymph nodes, *en bloc*.

But before treatment is considered, various tests need to be performed. Most important is the physical examination of the bowel itself using an instrument called a sigmoidoscope, which is inserted through the anus. Most tumours are close enough to the anus to be seen with this instrument. The sigmoidoscope also allows a small sample of the tumour to be taken away for examination under a microscope to confirm the diagnosis. There may also be special X-rays such as a barium enema. In this procedure, a liquid which is opaque to X-rays is poured into the bowel, so that the position and size of the tumour is revealed. Blood tests and other forms of X-ray can show whether any other organs have been affected by the spread of disease.

Though surgery is the main form of treatment for colon cancer, radiotherapy may have a part to play. Because the cancer tends to grow outwards into other important structures in the pelvis, some tumours cannot be removed because of the damage that would be caused. Pre-operative radiation, for two to four weeks, often succeeds in shrinking the edges of the tumour to such an extent that it becomes operable. In itself, such radiation is not intended to remove or cure the tumour, but to make the surgeon's job easier.

The type of surgery performed depends on the exact location and extent of the tumour. Hopefully, the surgeon can remove the tumour, and a portion of bowel on either side, and still have enough healthy bowel left to join up the two ends. The length of bowel that remains will of course be shorter, but a normal, functioning anus can be left intact. This allows the patient to control bowel action and so remain continent.

Where the amount of colon removed is large, there may not be enough left to allow the bowel to be rejoined. It is then necessary to close off the anus and open the bowel onto the patient's flank through a hole in the skin. This is called a colostomy (from 'col', for colon, and the Greek word 'stoma', meaning a mouth-like opening). Although many people find the thought of the bowel opening onto the skin unpleasant, the fact that this can be done is often life-saving, and it is important to remember that a surgeon will perform a colostomy only if it is in the best interests of the patient.

Recent developments make management of the colostomy very straightforward. A bag is attached over the hole; and many people find they can in fact learn to control the action of the bowel, passing a virtually normal stool once a day into the bag. With the use of proper equipment there is no discharge or smell, and the skin does not become sore. In most hospitals there are specialised stoma-care nurse who are expert in the management of colostomies and can help patients adjust remarkably well.

Where the surgeon thinks he may not have been able to remove all of the tumour, he will ask the radiotherapist to give treatment after the operation. This is aimed at eradicating any remaining disease before it has a chance to develop and cause further harm. Patients who have disease that has already spread some distance from the original tumour may be treated with chemotherapy. Some surgeons recommend the use of drugs during the operation itself, but others prefer to wait until the patient has recovered from surgery.

Stomach cancer

Stomach cancer is a common malignancy in the developed world, though incidence of the disease is now falling. It is found particularly often in Japan, Scandinavia, Iceland and Russia, but not, for example, in South Africa. Whenever such great variations in incidence are encountered, it suggests that some factor in the environment is involved in causing the disease.

Given that the lifestyle is similar to that in many other western countries, the incidence of stomach cancer in England, the United States, Canada and Australia is relatively low. The rate of occurrence is about one-fifth that in Scandinavia – around ten cases per 100,000 of the population each year. In England, the typical patient with stomach cancer is a man in his fifties. Men who are manual workers seem to be rather more likely to contract stomach cancer than men who are not.

Although some cases seem to be associated with existing conditions, such as pernicious anaemia (which is now very uncommon), there is no reason to think that ordinary 'peptic' ulcers lead to cancer. In most cases, the symptoms start as a new feature of illness in a previously well person. This is one reason the onset of 'indigestion' should always be taken seriously.

Like the lungs and skin, the stomach is directly exposed to elements in our environment – in this case the food and drink we consume, which often lie in the stomach for several hours. But the stomach is not simply a reservoir: it is also the place where the process of digestion starts. This in itself makes the stomach a remarkable organ: it needs to be able to break down the great variety of food that is eaten, and yet not digest itself. The lining of the stomach is exposed to change in temperature (if hot or very cold food is eaten), to any potentially harmful chemicals the food may contain, and also to substances which are formed from food as the chemical processes of digestion begin. For example, foods containing nitrates – which are widely used in fertilisers and preservatives – are chemically altered in the stomach to form nitrosamines. These substances are known to cause cancer when fed to animals in large enough doses.

There are many specific examples which support the view that diet contributes to the incidence of stomach cancer. In Iceland, the disease is comparatively rare in coastal areas, but frequent inland. A difference in eating habits between the two parts of the country seems to be responsible. On the coast, fish forms a major part of the diet, and is eaten fresh. Elsewhere, fish is preserved by smoking; and smoke contains high levels of hydrocarbons, substances which have again been shown to produce animal cancers.

Consuming large quantities of cooking fat in the diet is also suggested as a cause of stomach cancer. One reason seems to be that re-heating fat (which often happens when food is fried) breaks the substance down into potentially dangerous hydrocarbons, particularly benzopyrene. It is probably an entirely different aspect of diet that accounts for the Japanese having the highest incidence of stomach cancer in the world. They have a liking for raw fish coated in starch powder. This powder has been found to contain significant quantities of asbestos, which is a well-established cause of lung cancer when inhaled, and probably also acts as a carcinogen in the stomach.

Like many other dangerous tumours, the worst feature of stomach cancer is that it has often spread to other sites in the body before it is discovered. Usually this is by direct invasion of structures, such as the pancreas, bowel and the abdominal muscles. Blood-borne spread to the liver is also common. The way the cancer eventually draws attention to itself varies. But, typically, patients first consult their doctor because they have recently started to experience 'indigestion', a general ill-defined discomfort in the abdomen, and a feeling of being 'off colour'. Patients may also have lost weight and found their appetite reduced. These features of illness, though apparently unimportant, should never be overlooked and deserve investigation. Other signs of stomach cancer are even more imprecise. They include tiredness, which is caused by bleeding from the tumour, leading to anaemia.

The main treatment for stomach cancer is surgical. Wherever possible, the part of the stomach containing the tumour, and a portion of healthy tissue surrounding it, is removed. This is called partial gastrectomy. (Total gastrectomy involves removal of the whole stomach.) Both forms of operation allow the patient to continue to eat normally, though the amount of food eaten at any one meal may be less.

The chance of successful treatment is greatest when the cancer is small and confined to the stomach itself. One purpose of the tests used before an operation is to establish whether the disease has spread, and if so, how far. The barium meal is the investigation that is most frequently used, though it should be pointed out that the test helps in the diagnosis of many conditions, of which cancer is only one. The patient swallows a white solution containing the element barium, which is not penetrated by X-rays. The stomach and food passages, which are filled with barium, therefore show up clearly on an X-ray film.

It is also possible to pass an instrument called an endoscope (or gastroscope) down the gullet and into the stomach. This consists of a long flexible tube of glass fibres which allow light to travel along their length. The doctor can therefore see the lining of the stomach. A similar instrument enables a small sample of tissue to be taken for examination later under a microscope. Both procedures are easy and painless. The patient is not usually anaesthetised, though he may be given drugs to produce drowsiness and reduce anxiety.

Removal even of a part of the stomach is a major operation, and much of the doctors' work goes into assessing the general state of health of the patient, and how best he or she can be prepared for surgery. If investigations show the tumour has spread beyond the stomach, an operation is still likely to be suggested. Though cure is less common in this situation, removal of the tumour will prevent development of the most serious symptoms such as difficulty in swallowing, and vomiting.

Including radiotherapy in the routine treatment of larger stomach cancers has been found of little benefit. This is because healthy tissues near the stomach are sensitive to radiation and so limit the dose that can be given to the tumour.

Chemotherapy, generally, has more to offer. Systemic drug treatment can be used in two ways: as adjuvant therapy, or to control disease that has returned. Adjuvant therapy means that treatment is given even though no-one knows whether the disease is still present. Often, it seems that the tumour has been completely removed by surgery, and yet experience shows that in some people the disease will recur. So it may be worthwhile giving drugs to everyone who has had apparently curative surgery, just to be on the safe side. If the disease is going to return, its reappearance will be delayed.

The other patients who benefit from drug treatment are those in whom the disease is known to have spread. Cycles of drugs, used in various combinations, cause the tumour to shrink, and so prolong life. The exact sequence of drug administration is designed to have the maximum impact on the tumour, while keeping side-effects to a minimum. It is usually possible for the patient to remain out of hospital, enjoying a normal life between the cycles of drug injections.

So far, discussion has been confined to stomach carci-

noma, that is to tumours developing from the epithelial
cells that line the stomach. But there are other forms of
stomach tumour. The most common of these is lymphoma, a tumour of lymphatic tissue. Lymphomas can arise
anywhere in the body, but may appear first in the
stomach, or spread there from elsewhere. Although it
may cause the same symptoms as carcinoma, and can
again be a widespread disease, stomach lymphoma is
much more amenable to treatment.

To make the diagnosis, and remove the bulk of the
tumour, surgery still plays a major part. If the disease is
local, it can be adequately dealt with by local measures
such as the operation itself, and radiotherapy. Where the
disease has spread, chemotherapy can be used with good
chance of success, and around three of every five patients
who have the disease can expect still to be alive after five
years.

The prospects for better survival with stomach cancer in
general depend on the earlier detection of disease, possibly through some form of screening test. But the major
hope for the future lies with prevention. It is quite likely
that fairly simple changes in diet could avoid many of the
tumours forming in the first place.

Lymphomas

The lymphatic system in health and disease
The body has external protective barriers, such as the
skin, but its internal defence is the responsibility of white
blood cells, or leucocytes. These are of two types, called
after the appearance of their nuclei. Those which have an
irregular nucleus are the polymorphs. They are formed in
the bone marrow, but when mature are found in the
circulating blood. Their role is to deal with short-term
infections. The white blood cells which have small, round-
ed nuclei are the lymphocytes. Figure 7.3 shows the differences between these forms of cell.

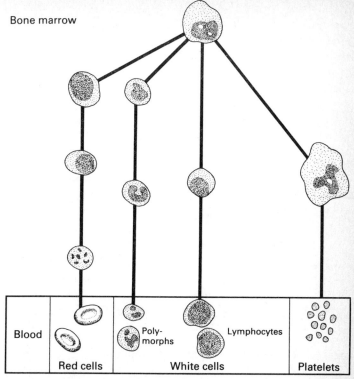

Bone marrow

Blood

Red cells

Poly-morphs

Lymphocytes

White cells

Platelets

Figure 7.3 The variety of blood cells, and their origin in the bone marrow.

Lymphomas are cancers formed by malignant changes in the lymphocytes, which form part of the colourless fluid – known as lymph – that circulates around the body. The lymph eventually drains into blood vessels near the heart, but for the most part is separate from the blood supply. The lymphatic system consists of a series of tubes, most of them too small to be seen with the naked eye, connecting the collections of lymph cells which form the glands known as lymph nodes, shown in figure 7.4.

The lymphocytes are key cells in the body's defensive immune system. They resist attack from infecting organ-

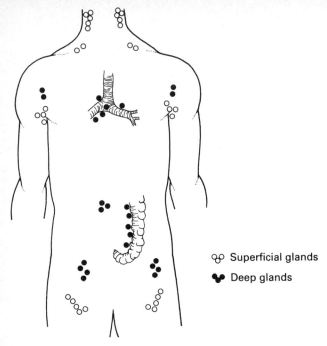

Figure 7.4 Where lymph nodes are found in the body.

isms, such as bacteria and viruses, and counter invasion by 'foreign' material, which can be anything from the tip of a thorn left behind in your finger to the poison injected by a bee sting. Lymphocytes also screen the body's own cells to make sure none has undergone a cancerous change.

Production of antibodies is one method the lymphocytes use in resisting disease. If you are injected with a small amount of the poisonous protein (or toxin) manufactured by diptheria bacteria, for example, the immune system reacts by producing a chemical antidote to neutralise the toxin. All foreign material (whether it is alive or not) entering the body includes chemical components that cause the immune system to react. These chemicals are called antigens, and antibodies are the substances lymphocytes produce in response. The process of immunisation ensures that our antibody defences are already in place and prepared to deal with any real infection that may occur. The second method of resisting attack is by activating the lymphocytes themselves. Lymphocytes can kill invading organisms such as bacteria, and also, under certain circumstances, destroy cancer cells.

But, like all other cells, lymphocytes can themselves become cancerous. When the normal immune system is challenged by a foreign antigen, growth of lymphocytes is stimulated. However, this increase in growth can occur abnormally, in the absence of a threat to the body. This abnormal reproduction of lymphocytes causes the lymph nodes to enlarge; and lymphocytes spread into other organs such as the liver, skin and brain. When the lymphocytes become especially numerous, they may spill out into the circulating blood.

The difference between lymphoma and leukaemia
To bring order into our understanding of nature, we try to classify the phenomena we observe. Diseases, just like everything else, are put in 'boxes', and labelled. But when we talk about lymphomas and leukaemias, our system of simple classification is in trouble, since the two types of disease are not clearly distinct. There are some conditions that are obviously lymphomas, and others that are obviously leukaemias; but many are in the grey area in between.

Lymphomas and leukaemias are both cancers of the white cells. When the cancer is confined mostly to the lymph glands, we call them lymphomas. When the malignant cells are in the blood, they are leukaemias. The cancerous cells themselves can be pretty much the same. What determines whether they clump together in the lymph nodes, or spread out through the circulation, are certain differences in the chemical composition of the cell surface which make them attract or repel each other.

One difference between lymphomas and leukaemias is in where the cancer cells are found. But the type of white cell that becomes malignant is also important. When the cancer cells are the polymorphs, they mostly remain confined to the circulating blood. Cancer of these cells represents the typical leukaemias, which are considered later. Cancer of the lymphocytes can produce either lymphoma or leukaemia, since the malignant cells can either remain mostly in the lymphatic system, or – especially in the later stages of disease – spread to the blood. But for the most part, cancer of the lymphocytes results in abnormal enlargement of the lymph nodes.

What is harmful about having too many white cells?
Uncontrolled growth in the number of white cells is a problem for three reasons. First, the cancerous cells infiltrate themselves into vital organs, and interfere with their proper functioning. Malignant lymphocytes that spread to the bone marrow can prevent the marrow producing sufficient red blood cells, for example. Those that clog up the liver and kidney mean that these organs fail to clear the blood of poisonous substances. Secondly, where the malignant white blood cells clump together, they form a mass which grows and interferes with the working of organs simply by pressing on them. Finally, although the number of white cells is large, the cells do their job only poorly. This means the body is less well defended against disease.

With most cancers, what we think of first is the actual 'growth' – the primary tumour, which forms a hard lump in an organ such as the breast or liver, and which can often be removed, sometimes along with the organ itself. What is a little difficult to grasp is that the lymphatic system is itself an 'organ'; but it is an organ which is spread throughout the body and which is composed of different elements, called compartments. The bone marrow, the lymph nodes, the lymphatic channels, and the cells that circulate within this system – all are part of the organ. The difference is that when one element becomes cancerous, it cannot simply be dissected out, as is possible with cancers of the kidney or colon, for example.

Signs and symptoms
Patients with lymphoma consult their doctors for several reasons, but often it is because they feel a lump or swelling – which is actually an enlarged lymph node – usually in the neck. In a normal, healthy person, it is possible to find nodes at the base of the neck on either side, around the place where the pulse of the carotid artery can be felt. These lymph nodes are especially prominent in children; and they become swollen during throat infections as part of the body's normal defence system. But in lymphoma, the nodes become unusually large, and remain swollen, despite the absence of infection.

When lymphomas develop, other symptoms may occur – including unexplained fevers, loss of weight, itching and sweating at night. Night sweats in particular are very characteristic. They probably occur because substances released by the abnormal lymphocytes affect temperature control systems in the brain. During the night, temperature regulation is re-set, and sweating is activated as part of the cooling mechanism. These sweats can be drenching, and often require several changes of sheets and nightclothes. Another curious symptom of lymphoma is that even small amounts of alcohol may induce pain around the enlarged lymph node. We do not know why. Neither do we know how lymphomas are caused.

Diagnosis
The only way to make a firm diagnosis of lymphoma is to remove one of the abnormal lymph nodes and examine it under the microscope. This biopsy takes only a few minutes and can be performed under local anaesthetic. If

a lymphoma is found, the pathologist can classify it into one of two groups. The first is Hodgkin's disease, recognised 150 years ago by Dr Thomas Hodgkin, working at Guy's Hospital in London. This disease occurs in relatively young patients.

Over the last few years, dramatic advances have been made in its treatment – so much so that the kind of medical text books found in the library are often out of date. Many doctors who are not cancer specialists are themselves unfamiliar with the most recent advances in treatment.

The second type of disease is called 'non-Hodgkin's lymphoma'. This may seem an unhelpful classification, but it includes a wide range of lymphatic cancers – and the only thing they have in common is that they are not the kind first recognised by Hodgkin. More precise labelling of these lymphomas is difficult because we now know there are more than 20 different sub-types of lymphocyte, and the differences between them are very subtle. Each variety can become cancerous. All of these distinct malignancies have a characteristic way of developing if left untreated, and may respond differently to therapy.

Investigation
Whichever lymphoma is found, the investigations used to establish the stage the disease has reached are similar. These include blood tests to monitor the circulating cells, measurement of the way the liver is working to make sure it has not been affected by the disease, tests of kidney function, and a chest X-ray. Levels of antibody in the blood will also be monitored. In some types of non-Hodgkin's lymphoma, such as myeloma, this is particularly important. Myeloma cells produce large amounts of a particular antibody, and this is shed into the blood in quantities that can be detected in the laboratory. Fragments of the antibody may also be found in the patient's urine. Monitoring the level of this antibody may accurately reflect the total number of myeloma cells present in the

patient, and can be used to follow the progress of treatment.

Computerised tomography is also useful in lymphoma since viewing X-ray 'slices' through the abdomen can often reveal enlarged nodes. Lymphangiography, X-rays of the lymphatic system, can be helpful; but this relatively uncomfortable investigation provides the same information as computerised tomography, and is gradually disappearing from use as CT scanners become widely available. A bone marrow sample will also be taken to see if it has become infiltrated by cancerous lymphocytes.

Treatment
Similar treatment is used for both Hodgkin's disease and non-Hodgkin's lymphoma. Except for the biopsy, surgery to remove large nodes is no longer used. Radiotherapy is remarkable successful in curing patients whose disease is confined to one area of the body, such as the neck or abdomen. Where the disease has spread more widely, so that radiotherapy would involve treatment of large areas of the body, drugs are used instead. This chemotherapy is also successful in many patients.

The staging investigations already discussed will allow a decision to be made about the most appropriate form of treatment. Some patients may receive a combination of radiotherapy and drugs. The particular plan of treatment used will depend on the patient's individual needs; and for this reason, few patients receive exactly the same therapy.

For localised disease, radiotherapy is usually given daily over a four-week period. In most cases, this can be arranged on an out-patient basis, without admission to hospital. The dose of radiation needed to destroy lymphoma cells is relatively low. But it is still necessary to ensure that organs, such as the spinal cord and lungs, that are particularly sensitive to radiation are protected.

When a lymphoma of the neck is being treated, adjacent lymph nodes in the armpit and chest need to be included within the area exposed to radiation. This gives the part of the body irradiated the appearance of a mantle, or sleeveless cloak, giving the treatment its name. When the radiotherapist is planning a mantle, he will make sure radiation reaches the whole of the tumour and its surroundings lymph nodes, while keeping radio-sensitive structures such as the lungs and spinal cord outside the radiation field. This is done by covering them with lead shields.

In the drug treatment of Hodgkin's disease, a combination of chemical agents is used (see chapter 6). Typical therapy consists of four drugs, two being given by injection and two in tablet form, over a period of two weeks. The two-week course, or cycle, is then repeated. Injections are given on the first and eighth day of the course, and tablets taken daily. Before each cycle, it is very important that a blood sample is taken to check that the blood-forming cells in the bone marrow have not been too severely affected by the previous injections. If they are found to be suppressed, treatment is either postponed for a week, or a reduced dose of drugs is given. It is usual for Hodgkin's disease to be treated by between six and ten courses of chemotherapy.

In non-Hodgkin's lymphomas, treatment is more complicated. These diseases can be divided into two broad groups: those that respond well to relatively simple drugs given on their own, usually as tablets, and those that do not respond except to a much more aggressive and intensive combination of drugs. Intensive chemotherapy often requires admission to hospital, and carries a higher risk of side-effects. These may include serious blood infections, and suppression of the immune system, as well as the effects described in chapter 6.

For both forms of lymphoma, the doctor judges the number of courses of drugs needed by the patient's response. Experience has shown that the best chance of eradicating the tumour is to continue until all sign of the cancer has disappeared, and then give another two cycles of treatment – just to make sure. Normally six courses will be given. At the end of four cycles, the patient is investigated using the same tests employed to stage the disease after diagnosis. If disease persists, treatment continues, with the tumour being monitored after every two cycles.

Most patients with Hodgkin's disease are now cured. But non-Hodgkin's lymphoma is more difficult. Though the lymph nodes can be reduced to normal size, the tumour may return. When it does so, the cancer can be treated again. In this sense, the tumour can be regarded as controllable, although it is less frequently cured. For this reason, as well as seeking improvements in chemotherapy, much research effort is being aimed at using the immune system itself to destroy the malignant lymphocytes.

Leukaemias

The marrow, contained within the hollow centres of our bones, is the vital blood-producing organ of the body. From it come three kinds of cells: white cells that fight infection, such as the lymphocytes discussed in the context of lymphomas; red cells, responsible for carrying oxygen; and platelets, which are small fragments of cells involved in the clotting of blood.

All of these cells (which are outlined in figure 7.3) have a very limited life. Red cells survive about 120 days, white cells three days, and platelets barely 24 hours. This means that the bone marrow is constantly having to replace blood components that are lost. With such emphasis on rapid growth, it is perhaps not surprising that cells within the marrow occasionally reproduce out of control – when the delicate mechanisms that keep cell division in check fail to function.

Leukaemia is a cancer of the white blood cells. To understand why it occurs, we need to know how healthy white cells are produced. It seems that the different forms of white and red cells and platelets, develop from a single stem cell within the bone marrow. This is their common ancestor.

Along each path of development, there are stages where cells divide. At each stage, they become more differentiated; that is, they become more distinct in form and more specialised in their function.

A cancerous change can occur at any stage in the production of 'finished' white cells; and one of the factors determining the kind of disease that appears is how far the cell has developed before it starts to reproduce out of control. But whatever stage has been reached, excess white cells eventually spill out from the bone marrow into the circulating blood. The malignant white cells also overrun the healthy cells within the marrow, interfering with the production of normal white cells, red cells and platelets. When the number of red cells produced becomes too low, the patient suffers from anaemia. A fall in platelet production prevents clotting, and the patient experiences nose bleeds and may cough up blood. Blood many also enter the urine, and bleeding under the skin can cause the appearance of purple patches. Inadequate numbers of healthy white cells leads to increased risk of infection. And abnormal growth of the malignant cells within the marrow may produce pain.

These are the general symptoms, and often the ones that alert the patient and doctor to the presence of disease. But there are four major types of leukaemia and not all have such serious consequences. Leukaemias are classified by the speed with which they occur and develop. Acute leukaemias appear suddenly. In chronic leukaemias, on the other hand, the disease has a long course of development, and in some cases the patient's life is little affected. Leukaemias are also divided according to the type of cell from which they arise. Myeloid leukaemia develops from the polymorphs, a form of white cell that is responsible for digesting bacteria; lymphocytic leukaemia is produced by uncontrolled growth of the lymphocyte cell involved in the immune system.

Acute myeloid leukaemia occurs mostly in adults. Examination under the microscope shows the cause is large and poorly differentiated cells (termed blasts) that form an early stage in the development of white cells. For this reason, the disease is also known as myeloblastic leukaemia. People usually consult the doctor because of anaemia and bleeding problems caused by the infiltration of bone marrow by the malignant polymorphs and the disease used to be quickly fatal. However, modern drug treatment now succeeds in eradicating the cancer in many cases.

In 1947, a drug called methotrexate was used with limited success in prolonging survival, though it did not cure patients of the disease. Since then, intensive research has produced drug combinations that are of greater benefit. The main problem is that these drugs are not selective. They affect cancerous and healthy marrow cells alike; and the dose needed to destroy all the cancer cells present is greater than can be withstood by normal bone marrow. For treatment to be effective, the patient's marrow has to be almost completely wiped out, leaving only a few cells from which the whole system must regenerate. This means that treatment itself is dangerous, and the patient has to be admitted to hospital for the drug combinations to be given. This is followed by a period of waiting, while the bone marrow recovers its function. Though many patients can look forward to long survival the outlook in this particular form of leukaemia is still not good.

Acute lymphocytic leukaemia tends to occur in children and in many cases can now be successfully treated by intensive chemotherapy. The disease makes itself felt in the same way as acute myeloid leukaemia, and the treatment is similar. But, fortunately, lymphocytes are more sensitive to drugs than polymorphs. The dose needed is less, and the number of drugs used in combination chemotherapy is fewer. Healthy bone marrow is not obliterated by treatment, which is therefore less dangerous, and the majority of patients can look forward to a successful outcome.

Problems start to arise when initial therapy has been completed. Malignant cells have been eliminated from the blood, but the drugs used – which are administered as tablets or by intravenous injection – do not reach the fluid that surrounds the brain and spinal cord. Cancer cells that have reached this 'sanctuary' therefore survive, start to reproduce, and threaten the body once again with widespread disease. The problem is tackled by injecting a drug directly into the cerebrospinal fluid through what is called a lumbar puncture. This involves inserting a needle between the vertebrae of the backbone, and into the cavity around the spinal cord. From here, the injected drug (usually methotrexate) can diffuse throughout the fluid surrounding the spinal cord and brain and 'mop up' any diseased cells that have found sanctuary there. For the same reason, radiation of the brain and spinal cord is sometimes used.

Chronic myeloid leukaemia develops not from primitive and rapidly-growing blast cells, as in the acute form of the disease, but from well-differentiated cells almost indistinguishable from their healthy counterparts which circulate in the bloodstream digesting bacteria. The disease is slow to make itself felt, but often becomes apparent because the liver and spleen are enlarged. (The spleen is an organ situated just under the rib cage, on the left side of the abdomen.) When the spleen expands, it can cause pain, which is severe if a small clot forms within the organ. Patients with chronic myeloid leukaemia therefore often arrive at their doctor's surgery complaining of abdominal pain. They may also have anaemia or bleeding caused by too few red blood cells and platelets. All of these problems can be controlled very simply with drugs such as Busulphan, which is given in tablet form, and can be taken for long periods. Busulphan is not very toxic, and most patients tolerate it easily.

The real problem in chronic myeloid leukaemia occurs after the disease has been present for several years, when a change may take place in the stem cells in the bone marrow. Instead of producing the specialised and relatively harmless chronic myeloid cells, they suddenly start to form blast cells of the same kind seen in acute myeloid leukaemia. This transformation moves the patient into the accelerated form of the disease, and is termed the blast crisis.

Although intensive chemotherapy of the kind used for acute leukaemia is often successful to start with, the blast cells eventually escape from the drugs' control and infiltrate vital organs. Much research is devoted to finding out why stem cells undergo their sudden change. Identifying the reason would not only help in the treatment of leukaemia, but also increase our understanding about the more general process of cancerous change.

Chronic myeloid leukaemia cells often possess a very unusual abnormality that can be seen when the chromosomes containing their DNA are examined under a microscope. A small piece of one chromosome (number nine) fails to appear in its normal position, but is found attached to chromosome number 22 instead. This 'translocation' produces a bizarre structure called the Philadelphia chromosome after the city where it was first identified.

Chronic lymphocytic leukaemia is a relatively benign disease which rarely causes death. Here it is the lymphocytes that are abnormal; and the difference between this disease and a lymphoma is not great. Lymphocytes have different functions within the body. Some circulate in the blood, some stay in the lymph nodes, and others patrol tissue such as the liver, brain and kidneys looking for damage and helping fend off infection. Malignant lymphocytes retain part of the function they had before they became cancerous, so the tumour assumes different forms, depending on the site of the malignancy. If it is the cells that occupy the lymph nodes that become malignant, a lymphoma results. But if the lymphocytes that circulate in the blood are affected, the disease is leukaemia.

Chronic lymphocytic leukaemia is often left untreated, provided no problems of bone marrow suppression or infection occur. Just as in acute leukaemia, the bone marrow can become infiltrated – but the advance of disease is much slower and less life-threatening. Many patients live to old age with no problems other than frequent visits to an out-patient clinic to have their blood count checked.

Cancer of the testis

This form of cancer is not as common as those of the breast, lung, stomach and colon. But cancer of the testis is particularly important because it occurs mostly in young men who have many years of family life and work ahead of them. There are few cancers in women which strike at such an early age.

Signs, symptoms and diagnosis

Normally, the first sign of the disease is a swelling of the testis. This may not be painful, and so is often ignored for some time. Eventually, the patient consults his doctor and is usually sent to hospital for the suspected growth to be removed. Although there are other causes of an enlarged testis, it is very important to start treatment of cancer early. Because of this, referral to hospital is a matter of urgency. There are few growths of the testis that are benign.

The affected testis is taken out through an incision in the groin, and not through the fold of skin, or scrotum, which surrounds it. This is because to cut through the scrotum may cause the local spread of cancer cells. The testis is removed together with the blood vessels and lymphatic channels which surround it. The cut ends of these vessels are then clamped off. The next procedure is the precise identification of the form of cancer involved. After the operation, the testis is sent to the laboratory for examination. Two major types of tumour occur – seminomas and teratomas. By cutting sections through the testis, the pathologist can discriminate between them.

The origin of the cancer
A normal testis consists of cells which generate sperm, and ducts along which these sperms swim. One type of testicular cancer, the seminoma, develops from the sperm-forming cells; the other, teratoma, arises from the more primitive cells that line the sperm ducts. Biologically, teratomas are unique – since the tumour cells can go through the same processes that are found in a fertilised egg. In this way they mimic the differentiation of tissues which should take place only within the embryo. So, inside a teratoma, it is possible to distinguish features usually seen in skin, bone, cartilage and glands. The tumour represents a bizarre caricature of normal development.

Certain teratomas, called trophoblastic or choriocarcinomas, contain elements that behave like embryos when they are implanting themselves in the mother's womb, and may grow extremely fast. A secondary cancer from this tumour, which is sited in the skin, can develop from the size of a pimple to that of a golf ball within a week. Fortunately, such rapidly developing tumours are extremely rare. But all forms of testicular cancer both grow within the testis and can spread to affect other tissues.

Staging and treatment
The last decade has seen a revolution in the way testicular cancer is treated, and successes in dealing with these relatively rare tumours offer promise for the development of more effective therapy for common cancers such as those of the lung, breast and colon. As with other forms

of cancer, treatment of testicular tumours requires that the disease is accurately staged. We need to know whether, and how far, the cancer has spread.

The testes' abundant supply of blood drains into large veins at the back of the abdomen, and cancer cells can spread via this route. They may also travel along the channels of the lymphatic system. The search for metastatic disease therefore has to cover a large area. The investigations used include simple X-rays, of the chest and any other regions where symptoms may have developed, a blood count to make sure the bone marow has not been affected, tests of liver function, and the search for substances in blood (called tumour markers) which are released by the cancer.

There will also be a CT scan to establish the state of the lymph nodes at the back of the abdomen and in the chest. Until this technique became available, many patients whose disease had spread were assumed to have cancer confined to the testes. This meant that they were not given the treatment that we now know to be most appropriate. CT scanning is one example of the way the introduction of new technology has been of direct benefit to the treatment of cancer patients.

After investigation is complete, wider treatment is considered. If no tumour is found outside the testis, there is often no need for further action. The patient is asked to return to the clinic every month to check that all is well. This is done by examining the remaining testis, taking chest X-rays, and measuring levels of tumour marker in the blood. From patients who had their testis removed several years ago, we now know that the chance of the disease recurring is highest in the first year. After this, the risk declines sharply until – by three years – the likelihood of a relapse is very small. For this reason, follow-up in the first twelve months is intensive, but becomes less frequent as the years go by.

If disease is found outside the testis, more treatment is required. The therapy used depends on the type of tumour, and the particular approach of the cancer specialist. When only small amounts of tumour are present, there is a choice between radiotherapy and drug treatment. Seminomas are especially sensitive to radiation, melting away rapidly, often within a few days of treatment. So, for this form of tumour, radiation is often preferred. But, in covering all the lymph nodes that need to be treated, an area right up to the diaphragm (the muscles that separates the abdomen and chest) must be irradiated. This large region contains a great deal of bone marrow – which produces blood cells. Radiation therefore risks reducing the availability of white cells, so impairing the patient's tolerance of the anti-cancer drugs that may be needed in later treatment. For this reason, many specialists now prefer to use chemotherapy at the start, even if the amount of disease in the abdomen is small. This is especially so in the case of teratomas, which are not as sensitive to radiation as seminomas.

Until 1975, there was little chance that patients with widespread testicular cancer could be successfully treated with chemotherapy. Several drugs produced regression of the tumour, but in most cases the cancer cells became resistant after a short time and grew relentlessly. Then, in 1976, Larry Einhorn (a cancer specialist at Indiana University) added a third drug – cisplatinum – to the standard two-drug combination that was in use. Cisplatinum is made from the precious metal used in jewellery by linking it to carbon atoms to form a platinum organic complex that is soluble in water and can be given to patients.

Combination of the three drugs, cisplatinum, vinblastine and bleomycin, dramatically increased the rate of complete and lasting tumour regression from 20 per cent to 90 per cent. Both seminomas and teratomas could be cured. Since then, the drug regime has been modified only slightly. For some tumours, vinblastine is no longer used. Instead, there is another plant-derived drug called VP16. The one drawback is that this very successful drug combination is extremely toxic. Both the patient and his family need to be aware of this fact, and of the details of the treatment.

To receive therapy, the patient is admitted to hospital, and an intravenous line – often called a drip – put up. A hollow needle is securely placed in an arm vein, and connected to a bag of fluid suspended over the patient's bed. Through a side tube, drugs can be injected – not directly into the patient – but into the fluid which is constantly flowing into him. This means that a variety of drugs can be given repeatedly without seriously inconveniencing the patient; this is important, since the full programme of chemotherapy takes six days.

There is another crucial reason for using an intravenous line. Cisplatinum attaches itself to certain cells in the kidney, where it can have a very damaging effect, and it is only by diluting the drug that these harmful consequences can be avoided. The patient therefore needs to be well-supplied with liquid so that the kidney filters a large volume of fluid from the blood. This dilutes the drug, and so prevents damage. To achieve this dilution, four litres of fluid must be given every 24 hours. It would be difficult to expect patients to drink this amount of liquid, especially if they are feeling unwell, and particularly if other effects of the drugs make them inclined to vomit. Use of the intravenous line bypasses the usual process of drinking fluid and having it absorbed from the stomach and gut, and so greatly aids treatment.

Patients receive platinum and other injections every day, through the intravenous line. During the period in hospital, fluid balance is carefully monitored by the nursing staff. To reduce the nausea that follows administration of platinum, the drug is given late at night, together with an anti-nausea injection which also helps the patient to sleep.

Some years ago in California, it was found that smoking marijuana reduced the unpleasant effects of chemotherapy. Not everyone liked the idea of smoking the substance, and many older patients took to making 'hash brownies' – cakes laced with cannabis. Research soon identified the ingredient that reduced nausea, and a derivative called nabilone is now widely used to combat sickness in many forms of chemotherapy, but especially when platinum is being given. Nabilone is effective, but does not induce the same degree of euphoria or pleasure as cannabis. There is no evidence that it is addictive.

After six days in hospital, the patient receiving chemotherapy for testicular cancer goes home, returning in one week for another injection. Three weeks later, the whole treatment cycle starts again: hospital admission for six days, intravenous fluids, and more chemotherapy. In total, four courses of treatment are given, taking three months in all.

The patient is then checked again to see what has happened to the tumour. If none is present, treatment is stopped. If there is still evidence of cancer, several options are open. One is a continuation of chemotherapy. Alternatively, radiotherapy can be used to dispose of the last remnants of the tumour; or they can be removed by surgery. The choice in an individual patient depends on where the tumour is, how large it is, and on the particular approach of the cancer specialist involved. Whatever treatment is chosen, there is no doubt that over 95 per cent of patients, even those whose disease has spread widely, can be cured using modern therapy.

After treatment, follow-up at regular intervals ensures that any tumour that might return is detected early and when small. Even recurrent testicular cancers can be successfully treated a second time with chemotherapy.

Current research is aimed at developing new drugs that are less toxic than the combination described; and over the next few years it is likely that admission to hospital for this unpleasant though successful treatment will no longer be needed. Several drugs are being developed that are closely related to platinum, but far less poisonous to the kidneys. It should be possible to use these compounds without the need for an unusually large intake of fluid.

Other clinical research is investigating the possibility of reducing the intensity of treatment for patients who have only small amounts of metastatic disease. A patient who has very small lung nodules, and no other evidence of cancer spread, for example, may need only two courses of chemotherapy instead of the four required in patients with very extensive secondary deposits of tumour.

Fertility

Dramatic advances in the treatment of testicular cancer mean that many men can return to a full and normal life. It is a tribute to this success that the question of their future fertility is raised at all. But it is a worrying point for anyone about to undergo treatment for testicular cancer, and needs to be considered.

One of the side-effects of intensive chemotherapy is that the sperm-producing cells in the remaining testis stop dividing, so that no more sperm develop. In most patients this effect lasts only a few months. But some men, especially those who receive chemotherapy combined with radiotherapy, become permanently infertile. Because of this risk, samples of sperm can now be stored in a sperm bank before treatment. It should be emphasised that permanent infertility is not the normal case: it applies to only around one in ten patients treated. With the development of improved drugs and ways of administering them, it is likely this problem will become less significant.

8 Psychological Aspects

The mind influences the body in both health and disease and a distinct area of medical practice – psychosomatic medicine – deals with this interaction. Cancer, its cause and treatment, is a key concern. So far we have discussed the disease as though it were merely a question of a fundamental biochemical error causing an alteration in the way cells grow. Cancer *is* that. But it is also more than a purely physical process.

There is evidence that attitudes and the way emotions are expressed influence the whole course of the disease, from the predisposition to develop cancer through to the effectiveness of treatment, the likelihood of cure, and the extent to which someone with cancer can readjust to daily life. By its nature, this area is difficult to research. It is not amenable to controlled study, and it is therefore hard to apply the same scientific standards as are used in evaluating medical theory and practice. But doctors are becoming increasingly aware of the importance of attitude and personality in anyone faced with the problem of cancer.

Who gets cancer?

With certain cancers, such as that of the lung, the most important cause (in that example, cigarette smoking) is clear and well known. However, even among people who develop lung cancer there are some who have never

smoked, have no family history to suggest a genetic predisposition, and have not been exposed to carcinogens at
work. There is no obvious explanation of why they should
have been unfortunate. This is the position with the
majority of cancers, which have no clearly identifiable
cause. We must assume that in these cases many factors
are involved; probably some are psychological.

This first became clear during the 1960s with a remarkable series of experiments on rats. Two groups of the
same strain of rat were separated and exposed to chemical
carcinogens. The only difference between the two groups
was that one of them was subjected to severe electric
shocks which occurred at unpredictable intervals. Rats in
this group developed a state very similar to the chronic
anxiety sometimes seen in humans. The incidence of
cancer in these animals was several times higher than in
the group not exposed to random shocks. Similar experiments have suggested that stress has a part to play not just
in the frequency with which cancers occur but also in the
rate at which tumours grow.

It is much more difficult to show that stress plays a part
in human cancer. It is clearly not enough to go to a group
of patients at a time when they know they have cancer and
assess whether they are more stressed than others. All
obviously would be.

The only way round this problem is to assess the personality of large numbers of people at a time when they
are young, and then wait for perhaps 20 or 30 years. By
that time a small number of the original sample will have
developed cancer, and the records of their characteristics
can be compared with those of the much larger group who
have not developed the disease.

There are now a few studies which have followed this
procedure. One, in the USA, has information on over
1,300 people who graduated from Johns Hopkins medical
school between 1948 and 1964. Since then, 29 of the men
in the sample have developed a serious cancer (skin
tumours, except melanoma, were excluded). This is a

very small number, but it is sufficient to gain an idea of the psychological influences that may be at work. Looking back to what they said 20 years ago, there is some evidence that the people who went on to develop cancer, compared with their peers who did not develop the disease, thought of themselves as less close to their parents. This may be an important result in relation to cancer since the same association was not true, for example, of people who went on to develop heart disease.

But the finding is still an isolated example. By itself, it does not mean much. However, it fits earlier ideas, based only on interviews with cancer patients, that lack of emotional attachment to an important relative early in life might be related to the disease. From the Johns Hopkins study, there is no indication that actual loss early in life of a parent, brother or sister has any effect.

At much the same time as the American study was started, Swedish researchers persuaded over 2,000 people to co-operate in a similar investigation. From it has come the suggestion that women who later develop cancer are more likely than others to refrain from expressing emotion when depressed. This again fits previous, but less soundly-based, ideas that inability to release emotional feelings is associated with cancer. Another American investigation, the Western Electric Health Study, has reported a small but statistically significant relationship between earlier feelings of depression and the development of cancer in later life.

These findings are only associations. They do not prove that personality causes cancer, and they do not suggest there is any certainty that a particular type of person will eventually develop the disease. The relationships that have been found are statistical. The differences they reveal are there only when groups of people rather than individuals are compared. And there is little evidence about how such personality traits interact with the causes of cancer we know about with certainty.

The idea that cancer has links with personality and

dominant mood has a long history. In the second century, for example, Galen claimed to find an association between cancer and a melancholy temperament. What is new is our increased understanding of the way psychological factors (which are very difficult to measure) can influence biochemical events (which doctors measure all the time), which in turn influence susceptibility to disease.

We can now be fairly sure that psychological events, such as stress, affect the function of the body's lymphocytes which form an important part of our defence against disease. It is also likely that psychological events influence our hormonal balance, which in turn affects the working of the immune system. Especially important here are products of the adrenal glands, some of which suppress the immune response. Stress in rats increases levels of these substances in the blood, and is associated with faster growth of tumours and greater susceptibility to viruses. It is likely that something similar occurs in man.

Adjusting to diagnosis and treatment

In many ways, the most stressful period is immediately before cancer is diagnosed. This is the phase of waiting and wondering: after a patient has gone to the doctor, and before the results of investigations are available. At this stage, all sorts of possibilities go through the mind; but cancer is probably feared above all other diseases. It is the uncertainty that causes greatest distress. Not surprisingly then, the actual news that the patient has cancer can often be met with great fortitude, providing the information is conveyed with tact and skill.

The facts about diagnosis, likely treatment and possible outcome should be given as fully as the patient desires. But people vary in their ability to take in details, especially at a time of emotional turmoil. For this reason, information is often kept to a working minimum at this stage and extensive discussion about diagnosis and treatment is left until subsequent interviews.

The diagnosis of cancer has a profound effect. Although some people appear to take it in their stride, they are a minority. For most, the word 'cancer' implies inevitable death. On top of that general fear come individual anxieties. Some people anticipate pain; others that they will have to undergo a series of unpleasant and degrading procedures or operations. Sometimes the precise fears are unknown, even to the patient, and can be revealed only with skilled help.

The main enemy, again, is uncertainty. A more complete understanding of what may happen can alleviate many of the problems, and a patient should never be afraid to ask. Often, fears can be shown to be unnecessary or exaggerated.

Nevertheless, considerable readjustment is necessary. What happens, and how patients can be helped, has mostly been studied in women having a breast removed. Here the problem is twofold. The significance of a tumour is realised, and produces natural anxiety about the physical consequences. But the breast itself is so bound up with sexual identity and self-image that its loss in many women is similar to bereavement. Almost inevitably, there is a period of depression; and these feelings should be expressed openly. Those that are suppressed may not be so apparent, but tend to be more protracted.

Since the feeling of mutilation and disfigurement is strong, and results in low self-esteem and lack of self-confidence, surgeons are increasingly prepared to consider breast replacement, either immediately or at some point in the future. This can be achieved either by insertion of an artifical prosthesis or by transposing a muscle from the back under the skin of the breast to maintain a more normal shape. The trend towards treatment which involves only partial removal of the breast is a great help. For many women, this conservation of their physical appearance can prevent or alleviate the distressing psychological effects of breast surgery, even though the diagnosis, and indeed prognosis, remain the same.

Surprisingly, the period of peak depression in many cancer patients comes not during treatment but several weeks after therapy has been completed. Patients are carried along with the momentum of events that surround the diagnosis of malignancy and the medical response, and it is almost as if there is no time for depression to develop. Later, when the immediate treatment has finished, to be replaced by another period of watching and waiting, the full impact of the disease sinks in. Being forewarned of this possibility may alleviate some of its worst effects.

As with depression from other causes, women who have had a mastectomy may find it difficult to sleep, concentrate and perform simple, everyday tasks. There are feelings of hopelessness and isolation, and the belief that they are being weak in allowing themselves to experience these feelings. The fact that this often happens at a time when the attention and care paid to them by others is diminishing only serves to exacerbate the sense of helplessness.

Several things can be done to make things easier. Recently, counselling services have been set up for the problems associated with the treatment of different forms of cancer. In the case of tumours that require a colostomy, a stoma therapist sees the patient before and after the operation. Many hospitals now have mastectomy nurses who visit each patient who is going to have a breast removed. One person who makes regular contact and can describe and explain with authority both the surgery and its after-effects can be of great benefit.

Half the colostomies performed are not for cancer, but for diseases such as ulcerative colitis, or following accidents. From the experience of all these patients it has been learned that contact with others who have had the same operation can help adjustment. Colostomy self-help groups are therefore also valuable. In the case of breast cancer, organisations such as the Mastectomy Association help by putting women in touch with others who have experienced the same problem. Stress and anxiety are undoubtedly reduced once the sense of isolation and uniqueness can be overcome.

Coping with recovery

There are patients in whom disease recurs many years after the primary cancer has been removed. The cells that constitute the secondary tumour have been present in the body since the time of the first diagnosis. Yet they make their presence felt only years later. This implies that the patient's body has been able to control malignant cells throughout the intervening period, and that something has eventually gone wrong with that control.

When a late recurrence is diagnosed, it is often valuable to try and discover why. In a surprisingly high proportion of patients, recurrence is preceded by some distressing event such as bereavement, divorce or an accident. This supports the view that emotional upset can precipitate the reactivation of disease and suggests there may be ways of coping with recovery that influence the likelihood of future illness.

Once the diagnosis has been given, and the intial momentum associated with treatment has passed, how do patients readjust to daily life? Some cope by denial. They put the whole episode out of their minds and pretend it never happened. One study which contacted cancer patients a year after treatment found that up to one in ten people claimed to have forgotten they had ever been treated for cancer. If facing up to the diagnosis is too stressful, denying, even to oneself, that it ever happened is an understandable defence.

At the other extreme, some people are so badly affected by the experience that they have difficulty thinking about anything but their disease. Fear of the illness cannot be overcome, and all their thoughts are coloured by cancer.

Most patients fall between these extremes. They cannot

forget they have been through a traumatic experience but do not allow it to dominate their lives. Some claim that an enforced reminder of mortality can be a turning point: an opportunity to re-examine values and achievements.

Professional help can also be offered during the period of readjustment. The first priority is to ensure that patients feel able to ask all the questions they wish, and that they receive answers which are as open as possible. Identifying people who seem to be experiencing particular difficulties shows where extra help should be concentrated. This can take the form of self-help groups of patients and relatives, and perhaps also nurses and doctors, who come together to discuss their common experience. Many value the support such groups afford, and a list of addresses is included on page 173.

Certain patients may benefit from specific therapy such as relaxation training, yoga or meditation. When properly taught, by practitioners who are experienced and aware of the subtleties of the area in which they work, these techniques can be of great value.

9   Alternative 'Treatments'

As orthodox medicine has become more technical, with its emphasis on complicated diagnostic and therapeutic equipment, it has seemed quite literally to lose some of the healing, human touch that used to form so basic a part of the relationship between doctor and patient. As procedures have become more difficult to explain, they have often been left unexplained. This loss of contact and lack of communication almost certainly underlie the recent upsurge of interest in alternative medicine in general, and a new enthusiasm for alternative treatments of cancer in particular. It has led some people to reject what is seen as a mechanical, 'conveyor belt' approach to care.

In part, and paradoxically, disillusionment has also been brought about by the success of conventional medical practice. It has dealt magnificently with the ravages of infectious disease; but so far has largely failed to 'deliver the goods' when it comes to the illnesses of affluence, such as heart disease, and of longevity, such as cancer. By enabling us all to live longer, medicine has also made it more likely that we will suffer these problems, to which it has not yet found an adequate solution.

At the same time as people have come to expect more from medicine, they have also become more aware. The old-fashioned, authoritarian stance of 'The doctor knows best; there is no need for you to worry about what is happening', is now clearly unrealistic.

This applies to all diseases, but especially to cancer. Where many of the conventional treatments available are unpleasant or disfiguring, and stand only a limited chance of success, the patient is obviously right to demand an informed choice about what is to happen. Sometimes the choice may be to do nothing; at other times to take only a 'gentle' approach to the disease.

The interest in alternative therapy is understandable. But there is little evidence that any of the suggested treatments work. Doctors are not so narrow-minded they they would blindly refuse to take notice of something that was of proven worth.

The alternative practitioners

Practitioners of alternative medicine fall into three categories. First, there are those who regard alternative approaches as complementary to existing medicine, and do nothing to undermine confidence in radiotherapy, surgery and chemotherapy as the main ways of treating cancer. Their aim may be to increase a patient's morale, or combat the symptoms of disease and the side-effects of therapy. For example, it is suggested that yoga may decrease the problem of nausea and vomiting during chemotherapy. Such help is welcome. Alternative practitioners of this kind make no claims that their treatment is curing the tumour, except by assisting that of orthodox medicine.

The second group of practitioners believe they can reduce tumour growth and perhaps even cure patients by special diets, encouraging a positive attitude to the disease, using herbs, electrical impulses, special healing powers, and so on. The claimed effect on the cancer may be either direct, or mediated by strengthening the body's defence mechanisms, usually the immune system.

Such techniques may help with symptoms, but there is little indication at the moment that they actually kill tumour cells. In our present state of ignorance, we cannot say that they are definitely of no benefit. But, as with any cancer treatment, the burden of proof lies with those who make the claims. There are histories of individual patients which suggest they have been helped. But what is needed is a proper study involving large numbers of patients and using some objective measure of whether or not a tumour has responded to treatment. At the moment, there is no reason for patients to feel they are missing an opportunity for cure if they are not also participating in alternative 'treatment'.

The third type of practitioner is the old-fashioned quack. Here, money is obtained for using time-consuming, expensive and totally spurious methods of supposed diagnosis and treatment. Quacks can practice in the obscurity of the small town back street, in fancy clinics high in the Bavarian Alps, or in a city's fashionable medical districts. Fortunately quacks account for only a small minority of the alternative practitioners.

What can be learned from the alternative approach?

A common thread running through alternative approaches is that the patient must assume some of the responsibility for decisions, and for tackling the disease. If this increases self-confidence, it is certainly helpful. Traditional medicine tends to 'process' the patient through a sequence of diagnostic tests and a particular plan for therapy – even if that plan is tailor-made for the individual. (The term 'treatment regime' itself suggests something imposed from above.) Anything that increases emphasis on the active participation of the patient is welcome.

Conventional medical treatment is sometimes impersonal, and unnecessarily inconvenient. Much of this is simply because of overwork and pressure on resources. But improvements could be made. For example, some hospital clinics have tended to give all patients appointments for nine o'clock, even though they knew the last patient would not be seen until noon. Having waited, the patient may be seen by a different doctor on each visit. If the patient asks for information, the answer may not be very forthcoming; and because of this there can be quite unnecessary anxieties. One case will make the point. Women who are having post-operative radiotherapy for breast cancer are often under the impression that treatment will cause them to lose their hair. In fact, radiotherapy of the breast does not lead to hair loss, and this should have been explained.

In the past, cancer patients were often kept unaware of their diagnosis, but their nearest relatives were informed. This led to people undergoing unpleasant treatment without knowing why. And the secrecy, often between man and wife, destroyed trust. The approach now is more frank, which allows honest advice to be given to patient and relative alike. But communication is still not a strong point of modern medicine. Many patients who receive the best possible treatment at a technical level may not have the opportunity for discussion which is essential in dealing with the emotional impact of cancer. The alternative practitioner is likely to see fewer people, and so is better able to sit and listen. Patients are allowed and encouraged to express their anxieties; and this can be of great benefit.

A feature of alternative therapy is that it claims to be concerned for the whole patient. Aside from general practice, medical specialties are organised around parts of the body, or particular diseases. It will perhaps be a radiotherapist who organises the overall treatment of a patient with a tumour, and it is reassuring to be in the hands of one person who knows a patient well. But if specific problems arise it is often necessary to refer the patient to other specialists. In terms of increased expertise, the advantages of specialisation are obvious. But they may be gained at the cost of making the patient feel he or she is a collection of anatomical bits and pieces and not a 'whole' person.

Part of the alternative approach is an emphasis on

self-help, and the aid, friendship and understanding of others in a similar situation. There is no doubt that someone who has had successful treatment can greatly increase the confidence of those about to undergo it. The same applies to coping with the side-effects of therapy, where it is important that patients know they are not the only ones to experience difficulties. People who feel they are on the path to recovery are better able to tolerate side-effects and symptoms. Hospital cancer centres are beginning to incorporate contact with other patients into their arrangements for treatment. But they are also learning that such groups need skilful guidance, since close relationships built up around someone who goes on to develop problems with recurrent disease can decrease the morale of the group as a whole.

There are relaxation exercises based on breathing, stretching and meditation that probably help some people cope with cancer. More formal disciplines such as yoga may also be useful, especially if they involve the close support of a teacher or counsellor in whom trust can be placed. There is opportunity for the strengthening of religious feelings, and for participation in healing groups.

Visualising the tumour and its response to treatment may also be helpful. To be able to 'see' the cancer, the patient needs to know the site of the disease, its routes of spread and appearance. It is then possible to visualise cytotoxic drugs coursing through the tumour's blood supply, and poisoning it. Radiation can be imagined, as it 'knocks out' malignant tissue, and white blood cells seen engulfing the cancer. Such techniques may be a help in withstanding the rigours of treatment.

Pain control can usually be achieved easily by drugs; and the idea that cancer means inevitable pain is totally false. Nevertheless, strong pain killers can lead to tiredness and a feeling of unreality. Techniques such as hypnosis and acupuncture are therefore being investigated as alternative ways of bringing pain relief.

Can alternative medicine cure cancer?

As far as we are aware, alternative medicine cannot cure cancer. In many cases, conventional treatment can. No alternative therapies have been shown to affect the course of disease. All the conventional therapies described in this book definitely do so, at least in a proportion of patients. That is the difference.

It is likely that some people having alternative treatment experience a relief of symptoms. The feeling that the individual can do something positive to help himself can also be of value. But there is no evidence that the approaches advocated by alternative therapists, such as changes in diet, affect the growth of tumours in man. Diet – specifically high fat and low fibre foods – has been implicated as one of several causes of malignant disease. And there is evidence that foods rich in vitamin A, such as carrots and cabbage, may protect against cancer. But we have no reason to believe that changes in diet affect the course of disease once it is established.

There are claims that certain enzymes 'desheathe cancer cells', so making them more likely to be destroyed. Injection of the extract amygdalin (of which more later) is supposed to have a direct effect on the nuclei of cancer cells. Tea made from the leaves of mountain box is said to 'prevent the formation of scar tissue when tumours have been dissolved'. And a host of dietary, drug and psychological interventions are held to increase the ability of the immune system to cope with disease. In some instances there is a grain of truth in these claims, in the sense that animal experiments have suggested an effect, or measurements of human biochemistry show some degree of change.

What is missing is the demonstration that any of these therapies actually have an objective effect on the course of cancer in man. Perhaps the immune system can be toned up by relaxation therapy, or diet. But that is not enough. It then has to be shown that cancer patients who have that particular form of therapy do better than those who do not have it. Such evidence is singularly lacking.

One of the most powerful arguments used by the practitioners of alternative medicine is that they have not been given a fair hearing. The answer is that it is up to them to prove their treatment effective, using the same properly controlled trials that evaluate new forms of conventional treatment. It is no excuse to say they are too busy curing patients to keep full records of the people they see, and do not have time properly to publish their results. If a person really does have a cure, it is irresponsible and unethical not to produce the evidence that will convince others.

Since alternative therapies may themselves be enormously elaborate, inconvenient, and difficult to sustain, it is likely that many who start the treatment eventually fall by the wayside. In at least some of the alternative therapies this leads to an element of winning both ways: if patients do well, the treatment can take the credit; if they do not, it can be argued the relapse was their fault for not sticking to the regime as closely as they should have done. In fact, people who improve with alternative treatment may well have improved anyway. Their improvement may even be the result of previous conventional therapy. In those who do not get better, the reason may have nothing at all to do with their failure to follow advice. To suggest that it has, is to add an entirely unnecessary burden of guilt to what is already a distressing condition.

One of the cancer self-help programmes widely publicised in Britain involves the consumption of 15 ground apricot kernels three times a day (the source of amygdalin), plus 17 other preparations of vitamins, minerals, enzymes and extracts. At the same time, patients have to adopt a diet completely devoid of animal products, salt and refined carbohydrates, and consisting almost entirely of raw grains, vegetables and fruit. After two or three months, it may be possible to reintroduce other foods. But, patients are warned, 'People tend to relax too soon.

Remember – to relax may mean a relapse'. In addition to 'eating for recovery', patients are urged to aid the detox-ification process by use of coffee enemas.

This entire physical therapy is then wrapped up in a programme of mental and spiritual exercises designed to 'present the patient with the key to the kingdom of change' and 'generate the subtle healing pathways of the mind'. A stumble at any of these physical or emotional hurdles can be used to justify the lack of success of the therapy as a whole.

Herbalism, the use of plant products, has a certain plausibility, especially when it is remembered that many drugs used in conventional medicine are based on care-fully purified plant extracts. This includes the anti-cancer compounds vincristine and vinblastine, derived from the periwinkle plant, and adriamycin which comes from a fungus. But the sort of doses and mixtures given in tradi-tional herbal remedies are not likely to be beneficial.

Spiritual healers, whether spiritualists or adherents of more conventional religious faiths, have not produced objective evidence of success. A medical panel at Lourdes assesses the cases of all patients who claim to have been miraculously healed by pilgrimage to the shrine, and there is as yet no case of a cure of cancer. But this is not to say that patients do not experience spiritual uplift by a visit to the waters.

Prominent alternative practitioners tend to be impres-sive speakers, and powerful personalities. Their publica-tions contain stories about individual patients, but no data on large groups, comparing the efficacy of one treatment with that of another. Their literature tends to name-drop famous authorities, or authorities that sound famous to those who do not have the information to judge. And the most dangerous mix plausible alternative practices with orthodox science.

It is often implied that the medical profession knows about these 'cures' but wishes to suppress them because they have an interest in maintaining things the way they are. Such a conspiracy is most unlikely. What could the reasons be? Conventional medical practitioners would be only too keen to offer a truly effective cure for those cancers that cannot yet be adequately treated. They would have nothing to lose, and much to gain.

The history of a compound called laetrile, or amygdalin (which can be prepared from almonds or apricot kernels), provides a good example of a substance for which great claims were made. But when subjected to proper scrutiny, the claims proved unfounded. Amygdalin seems to have been first described by a Greek herbalist shortly after the birth of Christ. In the 1960s amygdalin was patented and marketed to the American public. Twenty-seven of the individual states accepted the drug as being useful in the treatment of cancer, but an almost equal number banned it. This led to patients having to cross state or national borders to obtain treatment. Much emotion and profit was generated.

In response to public pressure, the United States National Cancer Institute evaluated the drug by asking practitioners who used it to give them details, including case histories and objective evidence such as X-rays, of their best results. From a total of 68 reports received, it was thought that six showed good indications of a response. This prompted a properly controlled clinical trial of amygdalin in 178 patients with advanced cancer of various types. Standard doses of the drug were given, together with the vitamin supplements, pancreatic enzyme and diet that enthusiasts for amygdalin claimed were also necessary. No evidence of improvement was found. The conclusions of the study were published in the *New England Journal of Medicine* in 1982. They showed that no patient benefited and suggested that, if anything, laetrile was potentially dangerous rather than beneficial. Several patients had symptoms which suggested they were being harmed by the cyanide products released by the breakdown of amygdalin in the body.

There are still people who advocate laetrile treatment,

and claim that the clinical trail was in some way unfair because it was conducted by people unsympathetic to use of the drug. It is difficult to see why anyone could have wished laetrile to fail. If successful, it would simply have joined the many other plant products that are in daily use in all branches of conventional medicine.

The fairest conclusion is that the various alternative approaches may be helpful in supporting cancer patients and their relatives. Self-help, and the idea that a patient should develop a positive attitude to the disease, and not simply become a passive recipient of a complex factory-like treatment programme, are beneficial. But there is no basis for making wildly optimistic claims that these techniques bring about cure. To do so risks wasting the patient's time and resources, and may cause entirely unnecessary distress.

The suggestion that people who offer alternative therapy are the only ones to practise a gentle or caring approach makes it seem that other practitioners are brutal and uncaring. This is an insult to practitioners of conventional medicine, who also respect their patients and are continually attempting to improve the treatments available.

10   The Future: Cancer Research on the Threshold

In 1971 the United States embarked on a National Cancer
Plan. Its aim was to find a cure for cancer using the kind of
massive, precisely targeted research effort that put a man
on the moon. Something went wrong. We still have no
general cure for the disease. True, there has been great
success in treating some types of cancer. This is especially
so with certain tumours of the lymphatic system and
testes, and with some leukaemias. In treating all cancer,
we now advance from a surer basis of understanding
about how normal cells work and how they become de-
ranged to form tumours. But these advances have tended
to come in a piecemeal way, owing much to good fortune.

Cancer research consumes vast amounts of money:
over £40 million in Britain last year, and many times that
in the United States. That we have not yet found a univer-
sal cure is not for want of trying.

Progress is being made in improving existing methods
of cancer treatment. The radiotherapy that is now offered
is much more precise and less damaging than before;
drugs that will kill certain kinds of cancer cell are more
effective; and we know a good deal more about the use-
fulness of surgery. But the major advances will probably
come from radically new forms of treatment, and these
are considered first.

Biological treatments: helping the body help itself

When a cancer develops, the cells have on their surface certain molecules that are recognised by the body's immune system as abnormal. This process of recognition is known as stimulation of the immune system. After stimulation, killer cells and lymphocytes act to destroy cells bearing the recognised abnormal marker. Almost certainly, many cancers are successfully prevented by these defences. But the fact that other cancers develop shows that the natural mechanisms of recognition and destruction are not always strong enough to cope. If we could devise ways of bolstering them, we would have a cancer therapy with great potential.

There are various ways of trying to increase both the recognition and destructive power of the immune system. One is by the artificial immunisation of the body with tumour material. Cancer cells that have been killed chemically or by heating are injected into patients. Under certain conditions this stimulates the immune system specifically to destroy any living tumour cells. Another method is to use vaccines that produce a general activation of the immune defences. But these kinds of immunotherapy have not proved particularly effective. Neither have the various kinds of lifestyle and diet, or even encouragement of certain attitudes towards disease, which are sometimes claimed to have a similar effect.

A third and potentially much more fruitful approach is to find the specific mechanisms involved in recognising and destroying cancer cells, and then selectively increase their effectiveness. We now know about several of the body's natural anti-cancer agents, of which the interferons are probably the best-known example. But there is also a group of molecules called the lymphokines. These include interleukin 2, the lymphotoxins, and tumour necrosis factor. Their normal function is to act as communicating molecules, stimulating and suppressing the immune system.

Interferon is a drug with public appeal, and promise. Produced by all normal human cells in response to viruses, it diffuses out of one cell and into its neighbours, conferring protection against infection. It is for this reason that the common cold, for example, is confined to the nasal passages.

The name comes from the capacity to interfere with the action of viruses, and the substance was first discovered in 1957 following the observation that it was uncommon for a patient to be infected by two kind of virus at the same time. Its anti-cancer potential was first suspected 20 years ago when laboratory studies showed that interferon caused malignant cells in culture to grow poorly. Experiments which followed confirmed that the substances could reduce the size of tumours in animals. But the difficulty of obtaining sufficient quantities of interferon hampered studies of its action in cancer patients.

The first studies of the drug in patients involved interferon harvested from vast numbers of white blood cells taken from the stocks of the Finnish National Blood Transfusion Service. This allowed small numbers of patients with very advanced cancer to be treated. Results with the drug were regarded as encouraging, but it was not until the advent of genetic engineering – by which bacteria can be 'tricked' into producing the substance for us – that large quantities of pure interferon became available.

This recombinant interferon has now been given to hundreds of patients, worldwide. The conditions treated include skin and breast cancers, and Kaposi's sarcoma, which is found in people with AIDS. The greatest potential seems to be in the treatment of a type of lymphoma, where 30 per cent of patients who have failed to respond to other treatments can be helped. It is likely interferon will be approved for general use in treating this disease by the end of 1985.

Targeting the cancer cell

The key to the cancer problem is to devise ways of destroying diseased cells while leaving healthy ones unaffected. This was the breakthrough which antibiotics
provided in the case of many infectious diseases: bacteria
were killed and normal tissues left unharmed. With
cancer, the problem of targeting drugs is considerably
more difficult since the tumour cells are derived from the
body's own cells and still have many of their features.
Nevertheless, on the surface of the cancer cell there are
abnormal molecules, and if a way could be found of
making a drug home in on these molecules tumour cells
could be selectively destroyed. In this respect, the recent
discovery of monoclonal antibodies is likely to be just as
important in medicine as the development of antibiotics.
The irony of this development is that it involves turning
the survival ability of a particular cancer cell against
cancers in general.

For 30 years we have been able to grow certain human
cells outside the body, in laboratories. All that is required
is a nutrient medium – usually derived from blood or
seaweed – which contains the right kinds of substances.
Many cell lines have been cultured in this way for decades. Given the prodigious growth of cancer cells, it is not
surprising that they survive very easily. It has been very
much more difficult to persuade 'useful' cells, such as
those from the body's immune system, to grow in culture.

An antibody is the product of a single immune-system
cell that secretes that antibody and that one alone. So it
ought to be possible to produce pure antibody by plucking
a single cell out of the immune system and cultivating it.
The difficulty is that antibody-producing cells die after a
certain very limited number of divisions. No way could be
found round the problem until Cesar Milstein and
Georges Kohler solved it, pretty much by chance, in 1974.
(The importance of their discovery has now been recognised by the award of the 1984 Nobel prize for medicine.)

Milstein and Kohler were trying to discover more about the genes that control the making of antibodies and stumbled across the idea of getting a lymphocyte from the spleen to transfer its genes to a cancerous bone marrow cell, termed a myeloma. The fused cell that was produced, and which came to be called a hybridoma, demonstrated that it was possible to combine the ability of a normal lymphocyte to produce specific and useful antibodies with a cancer's capacity for survival.

The hybridomas reproduce, resulting in an 'immortal' cell line producing a single antibody which can be harvested either by growing the cells in culture or by implanting the tumour in animals. Because the line derives from a single parent cell, which produces identical copies (or clones) of itself, the antibodies formed are called monoclonal. Though the work was first done at the Medical Research Council laboratories at Cambridge, the technique spread rapidly, producing a revolution in our ability to isolate and employ useful parts of the immune system.

High on the list of priorities is the development of monoclonal antibodies that will home in on molecules present on the surfaces of cancer cells. Such antibodies have great potential. Their first use is in assessing the amount of tumour present and in locating sites of secondary spread that are too small or inaccessible for detection by other techniques. This involves adding a radioactive substance to the antibody and then injecting it into the patient. The 'flagged' antibody concentrates in places where there is tumour, and shows up when the body is scanned by a camera that detects the distribution of radioactivity.

Such information is important in identifying sites where the tumour can be removed by surgery, or subjected to radioactivity. But the real prize lies in involving monoclonal antibodies more directly in therapy. One way is to couple a drug to the antibody so that it is delivered to the tumour, but not to normal cells: the antibody does the targeting and the drug kills the cell it becomes attached to. This is the old dream of the 'magic bullet' translated into terms of aiming and delivering warheads. Anti-cancer drugs in current use could be given in this way. But the precision with which substances can be directed to the cancer cell offers the possibility of using drugs more destructive than any that can be thought of at present.

One example is ricin, the highly potent plant poison which killed a Bulgarian dissident at a London bus stop in 1978 when an umbrella tip containing the toxin was jabbed into his thigh. The ricin molecule has two components. One part binds to a cell while the other punches a hole in it, killing the cell by preventing it from manufacturing protein. If the protein-inhibiting component can be isolated from the binding component, and the function of the latter taken over by the antibody, a highly efficient anti-cancer weapon is in prospect.

Laundering marrow

At the moment, the dose of anti-cancer drugs that can be given is limited by the tolerance of the patient's bone marrow cells, which are also killed by cytotoxic chemotherapy. A way round this problem is to remove a small amount of bone marrow, which is fairly easily done, give the patient a high dose of chemotherapy, and then return the unexposed marrow, which will then regenerate and replace what has been destroyed.

Unfortunately cancer cells have the habit of colonising bone marrow so there is always the danger that undamaged cancer cells will be returned to the patient along with the undamaged marrow. Monoclonal antibodies may have a specific role in preventing this from happening by cleaning, or 'laundering', the marrow before it is transplanted back into the patient. Ways of doing this include coupling minute iron beads to antibodies which bind to cancer cells. A powerful electromagnet is then used to pull out stray cancer cells before the marrow is returned.

These techniques are at the forefront of research into cancer treatment. But however striking the technical achievement, it is not enough simply to experiment with new ways of tackling the disease. New methods always have to be tested against the old. One of the advantages we now have is improved ways of comparing one treatment with another. This has already led to the revision of certain well-tried ideas about how best to treat the disease.

Surgery: sparing the knife

The surgeon's knife has been the traditional cancer treatment. But surgery now involves the removal of much less tissue than was the case in the past. Breast cancer is a good example, and the changes that have taken place are discussed in chapter 7.

A similar advance has been made in the treatment of bone tumours. Cancers such as ostcosarcoma and Ewing's sarcoma occur in children. The problem may appear simply as a pain in the leg, and the development of a slight limp. But although the initial symptoms are minor, until recently diagnosis of a bone tumour meant amputation of the affected limb above the level of the cancer – a disastrous event in a child's life even if it led to complete cure. New surgical techniques, plus the addition of radiotherapy, have allowed the development of surgery that spares the limb. Now, the tumour can be removed, together with a margin of bone on either side, and the tissue replaced with bone taken from somewhere else in the body.

In internal cancers also, apparently simple technical developments in surgery continue to improve the outlook and quality of life for the cancer patient. In the case of cancer of the colon, for example, the development of a staple gun has recently improved the surgeon's ability to tackle tumours. Before this advance, an operation to remove a colon cancer close to the anus required colostomy (see chapter 7). This procedure is still necessary in some circumstances, but use of the staple gun means that many patients are now spared colostomies. Having cut out the cancerous part of the bowel, the surgeon is able to reconnect the healthy tissue by stapling it together.

In this day of what seem like surgical miracles, it is often wondered why organ transplantation is not used for cancer patients. If someone has lung cancer for example, why not simply remove the diseased lung and replace it with a healthy one from a normal donor? The real problem here is the spread of the tumour. Although lung transplantation is a rare event, liver and kidney transplants have been used for patients with tumours in these organs, but they are rarely successful. By the time the operation is carried out, most patients are already suffering from widespread disease; the tumour has invaded surrounding tissue and set up secondary growths, often in distant organs. This makes a transplant futile, even if the patient's general condition is strong enough to withstand such a major operation.

New forms of radiotherapy

Radiotherapy can effectively destroy cancer cells. But, like surgery, this form of treatment cannot be ruthlessly applied. In the process of killing cancer cells, radiation may also severely damage healthy tissue. The dose that can be withstood by the lung, spinal cord, eye, intestine and bone marrow is much smaller than that required to destroy most common types of cancer.

Hope lies in enabling radiation to discriminate better between cancer and normal cells. Thirty years ago at the Hammersmith Hospital in London a surprising observation was made. The presence of oxygen makes cancer cells much more sensitive to radiation damage. Most tumours rapidly outgrow their blood supply, with the result that cells near the centre of the cancer are no longer well supplied with oxygen. This lack of oxygen, or hypoxia, makes them resistant to radiation.

Many ways of overcoming this problem have been tried. Though none so far has proved particularly successful, there is hope that modifications of these techniques will bring more benefit. The first attempt to make tumours more susceptible to radiation involved using oxygen under high pressure. A patient undergoing what is known as hyperbaric oxygen radiotherapy is placed in a cylindrical tube which looks rather like a torpedo. Such chambers are extensively used by divers to overcome the effects of decompression sickness. Oxygen is pumped into the tube at high pressure. As pressure builds up in the chamber, the concentration of oxygen also builds up in the patient's blood and tissues. The tumour therefore becomes oxygenated again and so should be more sensitive to the effects of radiation.

A disadvantage of this procedure is the clumsy nature of the apparatus, and its great cost. Results also are disappointing. Well-controlled studies of hyperbaric oxygen radiotherapy for a variety of tumours have failed to show any significant difference between patients treated in such chambers and those treated without them.

Another attempt at overcoming the problem has been the discovery of a group of drugs called hypoxic cell sensitisers. Such drugs, of which misonidazole is an example, behave very much like oxygen within a cell and so should sensitise it to the effects of radiation. The drugs are very small molecules which can easily diffuse even into the most hypoxic centres of tumours. Unfortunately, though hypoxic cell sensitisers work well in the laboratory, they have shown little promise in clinical use for brain and lung tumours and gynaecological cancers. A difficulty with these drugs is their unpleasant side-effects on the nervous system, which limit the dose that can be given. Newer, related compounds that are being developed should have less serious side-effects, and hopefully exert a greater effect on the tumour.

The lack of sensitivity of some cancers to radiotherapy is also being tackled by attempts to develop new forms of radiation. Conventional radiotherapy uses X- rays. But it has been found that other types of radiation, such as fast neutrons, deliver their energy in a way that is less affected by the oxygen content of tissue. The amount of damage fast neutrons cause is as great in cells and tissues that are poorly oxygenated as in those that are well supplied.

Unfortunately, fast neutrons are expensive to produce, requiring huge machines called cyclotrons. The largest is to be found at Stanford University in California, and the straight three-mile track of the cyclotron can be seen from flights into San Francisco airport. This was one of the first machines to be used to treat patients with experimental forms of radiation such as the science-fiction sounding proton beams, pions and mesons.

These new radiation delivery systems are attractive because they should have a great ability to destroy tumour cells that are poorly oxygenated. But all are extremely expensive, and all have practical limitations for therapy. The size of the angle of the radiation beam that enters the patient and the way in which the beam can be manipulated do not allow the radiotherapist to make a precise plan for the distribution of radiation in the patient. The development of new ways to localise tumours such as CT scanning has increased the ability of the therapist to see where a tumour is and where it is spreading. But the difficulty involved in determining an exact distribution of energy in these new radiation types limits the advantage gained by their ability to destroy hypoxic tumour cells. Larger, better, more flexible and yet more expensive cyclotrons are being built to overcome these limitations.

The increasing availability of computers has revolutionised radiotherapy in the last few years and will continue to have a profound effect. It is possible to obtain a computerised scan showing the exact location of a deep-seated tumour and that of the surrounding normal structures, and then use a radiotherapy planning programme to deliver the maximum dose of radiation to the cancer while exposing healthy tissue to the smallest possible amount.

New drugs: their discovery and testing

As we have seen, cancer-killing cytotoxic drugs are remarkably successful in curing certain relatively rare tumours. Unfortunately, patients with the more common solid tumours respond less well to chemotherapy. Theoretically, a drug that works for one type of cancer should work for all. But we understand only poorly how drugs act against cancer cells.

Cytotoxic drugs act by stopping cells dividing. But that in itself does not necessarily make a good anti-cancer drug, since there is a variety of normal tissues which also divide rapidly. As with radiotherapy, the need is for an agent which will discriminate between cancer cells and their normal counterparts. Unfortunately, it is unlikely new drugs will be much better at this than agents we have already, since cancerous and normal cells are very similar. This is one reason novel methods of targeting drugs to tumours by allying them to parts of the immune system are so promising.

There is a further problem with existing anti-cancer drugs: the tumour cells they are to act against have a remarkable ability to change. This mutation allows them to develop ways of resisting both drugs and radiation. An important example of a tumour which rapidly becomes resistant to drugs is small cell cancer of the lung.

Nevertheless, even with the drugs available, research can improve the way they are used. Drug combinations can be more effective than single agents, and a major priority is to make sure we are using existing cytotoxics in the best possible way. This means trying drugs in different combinations, orders of administration, and doses. It is also possible that different ways of administering the drugs, for example intravenously, orally or by intramuscular injection, may have a significant effect on the result of treatment. Being based on trial and error, this research is slow and tedious.

So too is a second approach – the development of new

drugs, which may be either versions of existing molecules, or completely new compounds. In the National Cancer Institute in Washington, a large screening programme has been mounted over the last two decades. Every new compound produced by the chemical industry is screened for its anti-cancer potential in a series of laboratory experiments, including tests on cancer cells grown in culture, and on tumours which have been induced in animals.

Those chemicals that are found to have promise are brought forward for development. One achievement of the programme was the discovery that nitroso-urea compounds (of which CCNU is an example) are of benefit in certain tumours such as those of the brain and bowel. But random screening for anti-cancer potential is very much a shotgun approach. It is research that lacks clear direction, and is again time and labour intensive. Only 1 per cent of the chemicals that pass initial screening ever reach the stage of being given to patients, even on a trial basis.

A more promising approach is to understand the biochemical basis for the development of drug resistance against compounds that already exist. Such studies are in their infancy. Assessing the effects of a drug on a particular tumour means that specimens of the cancer have to be obtained from the same patient before and after drugs are given. Most cancers are not accessible without causing the patient serious disturbance and such studies are therefore difficult to justify.

Within the next decade or so, there is not much chance we will find a new agent which marks a penicillin-like breakthrough in the treatment of the disease. The biochemical differences between healthy and malignant cells are too small. It is much more likely there will be a series of new drugs which have a small but worthwhile advantage for the treatment of particular cancers.

Demonstrating that new drugs are of benefit requires carefully controlled clinical trials. It is important to understand why such studies are needed, and how the interests of patients who participate in them are safeguarded. The first point is that all hospitals and research institutions have an ethical committee, usually composed of members of the public such as lawyers and clergy, as well as doctors from different disciplines. Before they start, all studies should be approved by such a committee.

Although a potentially useful new drug may be safe in animals, there is no assurance it will not have dangerous side-effects in man. So the first priority is to test for safety. Is the drug relatively non-toxic? Are there complications that arise from the combination of this new drug with existing medication such as pain-killers?

It would be wrong to involve patients who are likely to be cured with existing therapy, since the benefits of the new drug, though hoped for, cannot be certain. The first (Phase I) trials therefore take place with the help of patients who have very advanced disease, and little hope of cure. It is absolutely essential that patients give their consent in the full knowledge of the reasons for the study. Current frankness about cancer, and the prospects for survival, make such consent easier to obtain. Patients are told there is a possibility improvement may occur with the drug (otherwise such a trial would not be contemplated) but they know this chance is not great. Despite this, patients are often very prepared to co-operate in research which may later be of great benefit to others.

Even with someone who may be terminally ill, the major medical priority – first, do no harm – applies. The drug is therefore given at a low dose initially, and possible side-effects carefully looked for as the amount given is increased.

If it seems that the drug is safe, ethical permission is sought for a Phase II trial, in which its effects on the tumour are assessed. Since the benefit of the drug is still uncertain, it is used, with their consent, only in patients whose disease has stopped responding to other forms of therapy. Patients who have already received extensive treatment are less likely to respond to anything new that is tried. So these studies – by their nature – are biased against the chances of seeing any really large effect. This is part of medicine's cautious approach. But if the drug is going to be a worthwhile addition to the treatment of patients whose disease is in its early stages, some benefit should be apparent even in patients with advanced disease.

At this stage, it is vital to have a reliable measure of whether or not a tumour is responding. In the end, what we want to know is whether a drug can cure patients completely. But at this point, what is looked for is a reduction in the size of the tumour. Sometimes this is no problem. A skin tumour, for example, can be photographed and measured with a ruler. It is also fairly easy to follow the change in size of a shadow that appears on an X-ray. A biochemical marker, such as a protein that a tumour sheds into the blood, is also a good way of checking on the progres of the disease.

Even if the drug is effective, not all tumours – however similar they seem – are going to respond to the same extent. This is because patients differ in the way their bodies handle a drug, and because of little-understood variations in the molecular make-up of tumour cells. So each individual is classified according to whether there is complete response (when there is no evidence of the tumour after treatment), partial response (when the tumour shrinks by 50 per cent of its size), no response (the tumour stays the same size), or progress of the disease.

If an encouraging number of patients with advanced disease respond, the true worth of the new drug is assessed by giving it to patients whose disease is at an early stage. At this point the benefit of the drug starts to be measured in terms of the number of patients cured. Because most tumours that are going to return do so within the first few years, survival for five years without recurrence of the disease is often used as a standard by which to judge the success of treatment.

Since survival in any group of patients depends on their age, sex and the severity of the disease, we must be very careful to compare like with like. This means that patients given the new drug should be similar in all other respects to patients who were not given it. If we find that before using the new treatment only 40 per cent of patients survived five years, whereas 80 per cent of the same type of patients survive this long if they are given the new drug, we can be confident the drug is worth using. At that stage, the drug will become widely available.

The same system of careful evaluation is used if it is a new technique of radiotherapy or a new form of surgery that is being assessed. The process takes time, and effort. It is perhaps not surprising that people sometimes become impatient, and start making claims that later turn out to be unjustified. But the system of properly controlled clinical trials is the way currently successful forms of treatment have come about; and it is only by following it that we can be sure of having further successes.

Appendix 1
Reducing the risk of cancer

Many cancers can be avoided. For example, cigarette smoking is so closely related to cancers of the lung, larynx (voice-box) and bladder that there can be no reasonable doubt they are cause and effect. If there were no cigarette smoking, the total number of cancers would fall by about one third. The most obvious method of preventing cancer is therefore never to smoke; and – if you have started to smoke – to stop.

The danger from cancer can also be reduced by detecting the disease early. This lessens the chance the disease will spread, and makes successful treatment more likely. Clinics exist to examine apparently healthy people for tumours which are still too small to cause any symptoms. Take advantage of them. There is nothing to be lost, and perhaps much to gain.

There are also early signs that may be a warning of cancer. The list published by the American Cancer Society is reproduced below. If you experience any of them, you should see your doctor. Indeed, any new symptom or complaint needs to be taken seriously. All doctors would rather see many patients with minor symptoms that have no underlying cause than miss one patient who conceals a potentially curable disease for too long.

Cancer's seven warning signals

C   Change in bowel or bladder habits

A   A sore throat that does not heal

U   Unusual bleeding or discharge

T   Thickening or lump in breast or elsewhere

I   Indigestion or difficulty in swallowing

O   Obvious change in wart or mole

N   Nagging cough or hoarseness

Appendix 2
Glossary of terms

Accelerator, linear A machine used for radiotherapy in which electrons are accelerated by radio waves passing down a straight tube to strike a target. In this way high-energy X-rays are generated.

Adjuvant therapy Treatment administered after surgery as a precautionary measure, usually when it is uncertain if a cancer has spread beyond the site of the original tumour.

Anaesthesia Loss of sensation or consciousness. Local: in one part of the body, for minor procedures. General: when the patient is rendered unconscious.

Analgesic A drug that relieves pain.

Antibiotic A drug used to treat bacterial diseases.

Antibody A protein produced by the immune system in response to an antigen, a foreign protein which gains access to the body.

Benign Abnormal growths that are enclosed in a fibrous capsule and do not spread to other parts of the body (not malignant).

Biopsy Removal of a small piece of tissue from a patient for microscopic examination. It may be carried out by operation or by the use of a needle.

Blood count The count of the number of red blood cells, white blood cells and platelets in a sample of blood taken from the patient's body.

Bronchi   Tubes arising from the wind-pipe (trachea) through which air enters and leaves the lungs.

Cachexia   A general weakening of the body found in patients with cancer.

Carcinogen   A chemical that causes cancer.

Carcinoma   A cancer arising from lining tissue. This can either be on the outside of the body as in skin cancer or in large or small tubes within body tissues.

Carcinoma in situ   A localised cancer in which the cells show the appearances of malignancy but in which there is no infiltration of underlying healthy tissues.

Chemotherapy   The use of drugs to treat disease, especially cancer.

Chromosomes   Thread-like bodies which carry the genes located in the nucleus of every cell.

Colostomy   An opening for faeces constructed in the abdominal wall of a patient after removal of the rectum.

CT scan   Computerised tomography scan. A very informative X-ray investigation in which the combination of new X-ray techniques, together with computers allow 'slices' of the body to be seen.

Cyclotron   A machine which can accelerate electrons in a circle to produce very high energy radiation.

Cytology   The study of cells in body fluids such as urine or smears from the cervix.

Cyst   A small benign cavity filled with fluid.

Cytotoxics   Drugs used for the chemotherapy of cancer.

Differentiated cells   Cells that perform a specific function and that are mature.

DNA   Deoxyribose nucleic acid – the thread of life in the cell.

Endocrine glands   Glands which release hormones directly into the blood stream, for example the thyroid.

Epidemiology   The study of disease within populations.

Epithelium   The cells that line ducts within the lung, breast, colon and most organs of the body.

Gene One of a series of units arranged on chromosomes responsible for inheritance.

Hormone A chemical produced by an endocrine gland which travels in the blood stream and brings about its effect at a distant site.

Immune system The system responsible for defending the body against foreign invaders.

Immunotherapy The stimulation of the immune system to destroy cancer cells.

Invasive A growth that has penetrated surrounding normal tissues and is more likely to spread.

Laryngectomy The removal of the larynx (containing the vocal cords or voice-box).

Leukaemia A cancer originating in the blood-forming cells of the bone marrow or lymph nodes.

Lymphatic system The drainage system that removes cells and fluid from the tissues through the lymphatic ducts into the lymph nodes and recycles them into the blood.

Lymphoma Tumour arising within the lymphatic system.

Malignant Abnormal growths that are able to spread both locally and to other parts of the body.

Mammography The X-ray examination of the breast.

Mass A swelling or lump.

Mastectomy The removal of the breast.

Metabolism The process by which cells make and use energy.

Metastasis The spreading of malignant cells from the site of the original tumour to distant parts of the body.

Mutation Change in gene structure.

Nucleus Component of the cell that contains genes.

Oedema Swelling caused by the accumulation of fluid.

Oncology The branch of medicine involved in the study of tumours.

Palliation Relief of symptoms without bringing about cure.

Pap smear A technique used to stain cells from body fluids to detect early cancer.

Pathology The branch of medicine that studies the causes and effects of different diseases including cancer.

Placebo Harmless substance which has no pharmacological effect.

Polyp A small benign tumour that grows out of the lining of organs such as the intestine. It is connected to the organ by a stalk.

Primary tumour The original tumour, before any spread has occurred.

Prognosis Prediction of how a patient's disease will progress.

Prosthesis An artifical device used to replace part of the body that is defective.

Radical Treatment aimed to cure.

Radiotherapy Treatment with X-rays

Sarcoma Cancer originating from the connective tissue, i.e. muscle, fat, bone.

ScreeningExamination of a population to determine the presence of disease.

Secondary deposit A tumour arising at a distant part of the body having metastasised from the primary site.

Tumour An abnormal swelling or enlargement that is of no value to the body.

Virus The smallest known infective agent.

X-rays Invisible beams of energy which have been used successfully for the treatment of cancer and also for visualising internal structures.

Appendix 3
Drugs and hormones that may be used in cancer treatment

Chemical name	Trade name
actinomycin D	Cosmegen
allopurinol*	Zyloric, Zyloprim
aminoglutethimide	Orimetin, Cytadren
bleomycin	Blenoxane
busulfan	Myleran
CCNU, lomustine	CeeNU
chlorambucil	Leukeran
cisplatinum	Cisplatin, Platinol
cyclophosphamide	Endoxana, Cytoxan
cytosine arabinoside	Cytosar U
dacarbazine	DTIC
diethylstilboestrol	DES
doxorubicin	Adriamycin
fluorouracil	Adrucil, Efudex
medroxyprogesterone acetate	Depo-Provera
melphalan	Alkeran
methotrexate	Methotrexate, Mexate
nitrogen mustard	Mustine, Mustargen
prednisone	Deltasone, Orasone
procarbazine	Natulan, Matulane
tamoxifen citrate	Nolvadex, Tamofen

*may be used to prevent gout, which can be a side-effect of cytotoxic therapy.

Chemical name	Trade name
VM-26	Teniposide
VP-16	Etoposide
vinblastine	Velbe, Velban
vincristine	Oncovin

Glossary of drug regimes

Abbreviation	Drugs used
ABVD	Doxorubicin (Adriamycin), bleomycin, vinblastine, and dacarbazine
CAP	Cyclophosphamide, doxorubicin (Adriamycin), and cisplatinum
CHOP	Cyclophosphamide, hydroxydaunomycin (Adriamycin), vincristine (Oncovin), and prednisone
CMF	Cyclophosphamide, methotrexate, and 5-fluorouracil
COP	Cyclophosphamide, vincristine (Oncovin), and prednisone
CYVADIC	Cyclophosphamide, vincristine, doxorubicin (Adriamycin), and dacarbazine
FAM	5-fluorouracil, doxorubicin (Adriamycin), and mitomycin C
MOPP	Nitrogen mustard (Mustargen), vincristine (Oncovin), procarbazine, and prednisone
VAC	Vincristine, actinomycin D, and cyclophophamide

Appendix 4
Organisations involved in cancer help, education and research

---

UNITED KINGDOM

BRITISH ASSOCIATION FOR CANCER RESEARCH: c/o Paterson Laboratories, Christie Hospital and Holt Radium Institute, Manchester M20 9BX.

CANCER AFTERCARE AND REHABILITATION SOCIETY: Lodge Cottage, Church Lane, Timsbury, Bath BA3 1LF. Tel: 0761 70731.

CANCER RESEARCH CAMPAIGN: 2 Carlton House Terrace, London SW1Y 5AR.

COLOSTOMY WELFARE GROUP: 38–9 Eccleston Square, London SW1V 1PB. Tel: 01 828 5175. (12 branches nationwide).

HEALTH EDUCATION COUNCIL: 78 New Oxford Street, London WC1A 1AH.

IMPERIAL CANCER RESEARCH FUND: PO Box 123, Lincoln's Inn Fields, London WC2A 3PX.

INSTITUTE FOR COMPLEMENTARY MEDICINE: 21 Portland Place, London W1N 3AF. Tel: 01 636 9543.

LEUKAEMIA RESEARCH FUND: 43 Great Ormond Street, London WC1N 3JJ. Tel: 01 405 0101.

LEUKAEMIA SOCIETY: 45 Craigmoor Avenue, Queen's Park, Bournemouth. Tel: 0202 37459.

MALCOLM SARGENT CANCER FUND FOR CHILDREN: 6 Sydney Street, London SW3 6PP. Tel: 01 352 6884 (weekdays); 01 373 5861 (other times).
MANCHESTER REGIONAL COMMITTEE FOR CANCER EDUCATION: Kinnaird Road, Manchester M2O 9QL. Tel: 061 434 7721.
MARIE CURIE MEMORIAL FOUNDATION: 28 Belgrave Square London SW1 8QG. Tel: 01 235 3325.
MASTECTOMY ASSOCIATION OF GREAT BRITAIN: 1 Colworth Road, Croydon CR0 7AD. Tel: 01 654 8643. (1,500 volunteer helpers nationwide).
MEDIC-ALERT FOUNDATION: 11 Clifton Terrace, London N4 3JP. Tel: 01 263 8597.
NATIONAL ASSOCIATION OF LARYNGECTOMEE CLUBS: Room 26, 38–9 Eccleston Square, London SW1V 1PB. Tel: 01 834 2704.
NATIONAL SOCIETY FOR CANCER RELIEF: Michael Sobell House, 30 Dorset Square, London NW1 6QL. Tel: 01 402 8125.
SCOTTISH HEALTH EDUCATION GROUP: Woodburn House, Canaan Lane, Edinburgh EH10 4SG. Tel: 031 447 8044.
SOCIETY OF SKIN CAMOUFLAGE AND DISFIGUREMENT THERAPY: Wester Pitmenzies, Auchtermuchty, Fife.
TENOVUS CANCER INFORMATION CENTRE: 90 Cathedral Road, Cardiff CF1 9PG. Tel: 0222 42851.
ULSTER CANCER FOUNDATION: 40 Eglantine Avenue, Belfast BT9 6DX. Tel: Belfast 663281.
WOMEN'S NATIONAL CANCER CONTROL CAMPAIGN: 1 South Audley Street, London W1Y 5DQ. Tel: 01 400 7532.

UNITED STATES OF AMERICA
AMERICAN CANCER SOCIETY INC: 777 Third Avenue, New York, NY 10017
DAMON RUNYON – WALTER WINCHELL CANCER FUND: 33 West 56th Street, New York, NY 10019.

M D ANDERSON HOSPITAL AND TUMOUR INSTITUTE: University of Texas, Texas Medical Centre, Houston, Texas, 77030.

MEMORIAL SLOAN-KETTERING CANCER CENTER: 1275 York Avenue, New York, NY 10021.

ROSWELL PARK MEMORIAL INSTITUTE: 666 Elm Street, Buffalo, NY 14263.

USA NATIONAL COMMITTEE ON UICC: National Research Council, 2101 Constitution Avenue, Washington DC 20418.

MEMBERS OF THE INTERNATIONAL UNION AGAINST CANCER

ARGENTINA: Asociacion Argentina del Cancer, Tucuman 731, Buenos Aires.

AUSTRALIA: Australian Cancer Society, PO Box 4708 GPO, Sydney, NSW 2001.

AUSTRIA: Oesterreichische Krebsliga, Spitalgasse 23, 1090 Vienna.

BELGIUM: Oeuvre Belge du Cancer, 21 Rue des Deux Eglises, 1040 Brussels.

BOLIVIA: Fundacion Boliviana Contra del Cancer, Casilla de Correo 1406, La Paz.

BRAZIL: Divasao Nacional de Cancer, Ministerio da Saude, Esplanada dos Ministerios, Bloco 11, 70.000 Brasilia.

CANADA: Canadian Cancer Society, 77 Bloor Street West, Toronto, Ontario M5S 2V7.

National Cancer Institute of Canada (address as above).

CHILE: Instituto Nacional del Radium, Casilla 6677, Correo 4, Santos Dumont no 999, Santiago.

CHINA: Society of Oncology of the Chinese Medical Association, 42 Wu Szu Ta Chieh, Peking.

COLOMBIA: Liga Colombiana de Lucha contra el Cancer, Apartado Aereo no 17659, Bogota.

COSTA RICA: Asociacion Costarricense de Oncologia, Apartado 548, San Jose.

DENMARK: Danish Cancer Society, Solundsvej 1, 2100 Copenhagen.

EGYPT: Cancer Institute, Cairo University, Kasr El Aini Street, Fom El Kalig, Cairo.

FEDERAL REPUBLIC OF GERMANY: Deutsche Krebs-gesellschaft e. V., Hufelandstrasse 55, 4300 Essen--Holsterhausen.

Deutsches Krebsforschungszentrum, Im Neuenheimer Feld 280, Postfach 101949, 6900 Heidelberg 1.

FINLAND: Suomen Syopayhdistys, Liisankatu 21B, 00170 Helsinki 17.

FRANCE: Fondation Curie, 26 Rue d'Ulm, 75231 Paris Cedex 05.

Lique Nationale Française contre le Cancer, 90 Rue d'Assas, 75006 Paris.

GREECE: Hellenic Cancer Society, 6 George Street, Kanigos Square, Athens 141.

HONG KONG: The Hong Kong Anti-Cancer Society, Brick Hill, Aberdeen

ICELAND: The Icelandic Cancer Society, PO Box 523, Reykjavik.

INDIA: Indian Cancer Society, Dr Ernest Borges Marg, Parel, Bombay 400012.

Tata Memorial Centre (address as above).

INDONESIA: Indonesian Cancer Society, J1. Jendral S. Parman 82, Slipi, Djakarta.

IRELAND: Irish Cancer Society, 5 Northumberland Road, Dublin 4.

ISRAEL: Israel Cancer Association, PO Box 7065, Tel-Aviv.

ITALY: Istituto Nazionale per lo Studio e la Cura dei Tumori, Via Venezian 1, 20133 Milan.

Lega Italiana per la Lotta contro i Tumori, Via Alessandro Torlonia 15, 00161 Rome.

JAMAICA: Ministry of Health and Environmental Control, 21 Slipe Pen Road, PO Box 478, Kingston.

JAPAN: Japan Cancer Society, 7th floor, Asahi Shimbun Building, Yuraku-Cho, Chiyoda-ku, Tokyo 170.

Japanese Foundation for Cancer Research, c/o Cancer Institute, Kami-Ikebukuro 1–37–1, Toshima-ku, Tokyo.

JORDAN: Ministry of Health, PO Box 86, Amman.

KENYA: Cancer Council of Kenya, PO Box 40563, Nairobi.

KOREA: Korean Cancer Society, Chung Ang Hospital, 161 Waryong Dong, Chongno-Gu, Seoul 110.

KUWAIT: Ministry of Public Health, PO Box 5, Kuwait.

MALAYSIA: National Cancer Society of Malaysia, PO Box 2187, Kuala Lumpur.

MEXICO: Instituto Nacional de Cancerologia, Av Ninos Heroes 151, Mexico City 7.

NETHERLANDS: Konigin Wilhlemina Fonds – Nederlandse Organisatie voor de Kankerbestrijding, de Lairessestraat 33, Amsterdam.

NEW ZEALAND: Cancer Society of New Zealand, PO Box 10340, Wellington C1.

NORWAY: Norwegian Cancer Society, Huitfeldtsgt 49, Oslo 2.

Norwegian Society for Fighting Cancer, Kongenst 6, Oslo 1.

PERU: Liga Peruana de Lucha contra el Cancer, Jr Chancay 922 Of 1, Lima.

PHILIPPINES: Phillippine Cancer Society, 310 San Rafael, PO Box 3066, Manila 2800.

PORTUGAL: Liga Portuguesa contra o Cancro, rua Prof Edmundo Lima Basto, Lisbon 4.

SINGAPORE: The Singapore Cancer Society, 334 Peace Centre 1, Sophia Road, Singapore 9.

SOUTH AFRICA: The National Cancer Association of South Africa, PO Box 2000, Johannesburg.

SPAIN: Asociacion Espanola contra el Cancer, Amador de los Rios 5, Madrid 4.

SWEDEN: The Cancer Society of Stockholm, Radium-hemmet, 104 01 Stockholm..

The Swedish Cancer Society, Sturegatan 14, 114 36 Stockholm.

SWITZERLAND: Schweizerische Krebsliga, Baumlein-gasse 22, 4001 Basle.

THAILAND: Thai Cancer Society, 1909/86 Soi Ruam Patana, Charunsanitwong Road, Bangplud, Bankoknoi, Dhonburi.

TRINIDAD: The Trinidad and Tobago Cancer Society, 95 Mucurapo Road, St James, Cocorite.

TURKEY: National Federation against Cancer, Lobut Sok 61, Sishane, Istanbul.

VENEZUELA: Sociedad Anticanceros de Venezuela, Apartado de Correos 6702, Canonigos a Esperanza 43, Carcacas 101.

Index